Incremental Structures and Wear Patterns of Teeth for Age Assessment of Red Deer

Tina Dudley Furniss-Roe

BAR International Series 1835
2008

This title published by

Archaeopress
Publishers of British Archaeological Reports
Gordon House
276 Banbury Road
Oxford OX2 7ED
England
bar@archaeopress.com
www.archaeopress.com

BAR S1835

Incremental Structures and Wear Patterns of Teeth for Age Assessment of Red Deer

ISBN 978 1 4073 0319 2

Printed in England by Alden HenDi, Oxfordshire

All BAR titles are available from:

Hadrian Books Ltd
122 Banbury Road
Oxford
OX2 7BP
England
bar@hadrianbooks.co.uk

The current BAR catalogue with details of all titles in print, prices and means of payment is available free from Hadrian Books or may be downloaded from www.archaeopress.com

Acknowledgements

There are a number of people and institutions without whom this thesis would not have been possible:

Hugh Rose of the British Deer Society, who supplied jaws from both England and Scotland, who gave me the benefit of his encyclopedic knowledge of deer and put me in contact with many others in the deer world. His enthusiasm was catching; The Deer Commission for Scotland, and in particular Colin McLean who provided the known aged material and hundreds of other jaws from around Scotland; Barry Brown, who provided invaluable advice on dental anatomy, photography, and scoring schemes, and acted as a second examiner of incremental structures; Toby Hall, who facilitated the mathematics and statistics and David Downham; Norma Chapman, who supplied known aged material from Richmond Park; Ian Chaplin of Buehler and Ben Harris without whose expertise in thin sectioning I would not have been able to begin.

I must thank my supervisor Professor Paul Mellars, for suggesting such an interesting field of research, and for his support throughout. I am very grateful to the NERC for funding. I am also very grateful to all the estates and the game keepers, rangers, and stalkers who collected deer jaws for me: these include Des Dugan, Sandy Masson, Peter Ord, Mr Pall, J. Mayfield, and many, many more. I would also like to express my thanks to Professor Tim Clutton-Brock and Fiona Guinness for allowing me access to their collection of known aged Red deer material from Rum.

I benefited scientifically from the advice and conversation of Anne Pike-Tay, Rob Foley, Margaret Belattie, Geoff Bailey, Ariane Burke, Margaret Beasley, Nicky Milner, Daniel Lieberman, Marsha Levine, Sebastian Payne, Davina Hoile, and Michael Baxter-Brown. I have also benefited, through the mediation of Barry Brown, from the advice of Alan Boyde and Sheila Jones.

A very pleasant and supportive working environment with excellent facilities was provided by the Department of Archaeology of the University of Cambridge, and by the McDonald Institute for Archaeological Research. In this regard I would particularly like to thank Charlie French, Chris Scarre, Jessica Rippengal, Julie Boast, Colin Lomas, and Melanie Leggatt.

I also received valuable technical advice from Patsy Whelehan on X rays, Neil Brodie on computer image enhancement, Gwil Owen on photography, and Rod Long on the production of casts. The excellent illustrations in this thesis were drawn by Sandra Doyle and Anita Pounder.

I am grateful to David Davison of Archaeopress for his support.

Thanks also to my many friends, particularly Hugh and Margie Rose for their constant support, inspiration and hospitality; Norma Chapman for her friendship and support; Toby Hall for all his amazing encouragement, stimulation and tireless commitment; Barry Brown, who taught me so much about teeth and life, and who never stopped believing; Claudine Brown for her continued support Anita Pounder and Beryl Lott for their understanding; and Neil Brodie for his constant nagging while keeping me smiling throughout; John Beard for being such an understanding boss when I was attempting to combine full time work with writing up.

Finally, deepest thanks and sincere gratitude are due to my family and friends for their love, understanding, patience and encouragement to bring this thesis to publication, particularly my husband Robert.

With such a wealth of professional and friendly help at my disposal, it only remains for me to acknowledge that any mistakes within this book are my own.

Contents

List of Figures

List of Tables

Introduction

The ability to age animals accurately is of great importance both to archaeologists and to wildlife managers. Archaeologists are also particularly interested in the ability to determine the season of death of mammals, in order to reach a greater understanding of how man was exploiting or responding to his environment. A number of methods of age determination are available to wildlife managers, who have the advantage of having an entire animal in good condition at their disposal. Archaeologists, however, have more limited resources, and often wish to attempt age, and even seasonality, assessments using only bones and teeth. Teeth survive very well in the ground, and can often reveal information that would otherwise be lost, such as the species, which were available, and whether they were being hunted, scavenged, or farmed.

Incremental analysis is based on the appositional growth of cementum, which is laid down on the outside of the tooth roots throughout the life of an animal. It is widely conjectured that, broadly speaking, one narrow *line* and one wider *band* are laid down during each year of life. If this conjecture is valid, then it should be possible to determine the age of the animal by counting this pair of lines and bands. Taking the conjecture a step further, it is also believed by many that the lines are laid down in winter and the bands in summer: thus the season of death can be identified by observing whether the outermost layer is a line or a band. If these conjectures were true, and if the technical process of identifying and counting increments were possible, then cementum incremental analysis would provide a remarkable working tool for archaeologists, enabling them accurately to determine the seasonal usage of sites. With this in mind, the principal aim of this research was to examine the scientific basis and methodology of incremental analysis in order to arrive at increased understanding of the British Mesolithic.

This technique has been used by wildlife biologists for over 60 years as a means of obtaining accurate age estimates of many species of wild animals. It is only more recently that it has been adopted by archaeologists (Saxon and Higham 1968). In the following thirty years, a plethora of techniques for sectioning and interpreting bands, lines, layers, growth zones, annuli, increments, rest lines, and summer and winter bands have been proposed.

The aim of this thesis, then, was to examine every aspect of incremental analysis: the scientific basis, the methodology of thin section production, microscopical techniques, and interpretation, in order to obtain the greatest possible amount of information from a rather specialised technique. The species chosen was Red deer, a common animal on archaeological sites in British prehistory.

A large modern control sample, including many of known age and date of death, was examined meticulously, with every care being taken to produce high quality thin sections and to examine them in as many different ways as possible. As the research progressed, it became clear that, at least using standard ground thin sections (a necessary restriction if the method is to be applied to archaeological samples which do not withstand decalcification), there are very serious obstacles to obtaining accurate age assessments of Red deer, let alone seasonality determination.

There are a number of reasons for the lack of success of the method, each of which is treated in some detail in the thesis. Amongst the most important are:

1. Cementum is dynamic, and is not distributed evenly around the tooth root.
2. Interpretation of incremental structures in cementum has a high subjective component, and a trained examiner cannot reliably replicate his measurements on a given sample when it is examined independently on different occasions.
3. The causal factors giving rise to cementum layering have yet to be identified; and although there is no doubt that an incremental structure is present, it has not been possible to assign them with any certainty to seasons.
4. Sectioning techniques can give rise to errors in interpretation.
5. Incremental analysis is expensive and time-consuming, requires specialist training and specialist equipment for thin section production and analysis. In the archaeological context, it also involves the destruction of valuable specimens.
6. Cementum can be damaged and modified by a number of influences, both before and after the death of the animal.

It does, however, seem possible to achieve approximate ageing from thick sections of teeth, although these are certainly not suitable for seasonality determination.

Once it had been established that there are inherent obstacles to the application of incremental analysis, it was decided to attempt to derive a more accurate and reliable means of ageing Red deer using tooth wear. In the second part of the thesis a new scoring scheme is motivated, derived, and tested, and is shown to be both more accurate and much more reliable than cementum incremental analysis. Since tooth wear analysis is inexpensive, relatively quick, requires little training, and does not destroy the specimen under examination, it seems sensible that this method, rather than incremental analysis, should be used for building up age profiles on archaeological sites.

Chapter One
The structure and function of cementum

It is recognized (see, for example, Thomas and Bandy 1975, Lieberman & Meadow 1992) that, in order to determine whether or not the age and season of death of an animal can be established by means of cementum increments, it is imperative to have a detailed understanding of the nature of cementum: how it is formed, its composition and structure, its function, the changes which it may undergo, and the factors which influence its incremental deposition. Despite this, very few archaeologists engaged in this area of research have made a serious attempt to understand the biology of cementum and its implications for the analysis of incremental layers. According to Lieberman (1990, 1994), one of the primary reasons that incremental analysis is not more widespread among archaeologists is their lack of understanding of the causes of cementum layering. While agreeing with his conclusion, it should also be pointed out that this lack of understanding is not confined to archaeologists - dental anatomists also disagree about many aspects of this, the "least-known mineralized tissue" (Bosshardt and Schroeder 1996): cementum is a complex tissue which is constantly changing. However, in many instances, archaeological material has been sectioned by researchers who seem to have so little understanding of the substance they are studying that their results must be regarded with skepticism. Most archaeological work has as its basis one or more of the following assumptions:

a) That incremental layers are always to be seen, and are laid down at a constant rate.
b) That incremental layers are always seasonal, and follow a uniform annual rhythm.
c) That cementum, having been laid down, is not subject to change.
d) That the same number of incremental layers are to be found at any location on the tooth root (often it is not stated which location has been analyzed), and
e) That interpretative methods developed for one species are applicable to others.

All of these assumptions have been disputed. In order to resolve such disputes, it is necessary not only to have a large modern control sample for each species under consideration, but also to understand the mechanism of cementum formation.

In this chapter I shall review the structure of cementum; discuss some of the prevailing theories regarding its function, and the possible changes (such as resorption) which could affect it, thereby leading to discrepancies in incremental analysis; and discuss theories regarding the causes of incremental layering within cementum. To provide a framework for a detailed discussion of cementum, it is necessary first to describe briefly the structure of teeth as a whole.

1. THE STRUCTURE OF TEETH

To function properly teeth need to be securely anchored, to be harder than the food that they are cutting and grinding, and to be able to withstand the stress placed on them by constant pressure of mastication (eating, grinding).

Teeth are held into bone sockets in the jaw bone (the alveoli) by periodontal ligament attached to the cementum which surrounds the roots, the areas of the tooth below the gum line that hold the tooth in place. Klevezal (1996) makes the distinction between growth patterns in teeth in evergrowing and non-evergrowing teeth. Non-evergrowing teeth have distinguished crown and roots, and are found in most mammals (Klevezal 1996). In mature mammals, the area of the tooth covered by enamel above the bone and projecting into the mouth is generally called the crown. The coronal end of the tooth is the top of the crown, while the apex is the very bottom point of the root. In some teeth there are infoldings within the body of the crown, down from the occlusal surface (the area of the tooth that faces the teeth in the opposite jaw) and these are called infundibula (Hillson 1986).

Evergrowing teeth do not form genuine roots. At the base of the tooth there is a growth zone providing constant formation of dentine, cementum and enamel to ensure the constant length of the tooth as it responds to permanent wear at the apex. This type of tooth is found in the incisors of rodents and some primates (Klevezal 1996).

Teeth have five main components: enamel, dentine, pulp, cementum, and the periodontal ligament. These are briefly described in turn below.

Enamel is the external tissue of the crown, the area of the tooth that usually protrudes into the mouth. It is made up of a crystalline structure and is almost entirely inorganic (Hillson 1986). It is the most highly calcified and hardest tissue of the body (Scott and Symons 1974). It is almost pure (96%) mineral (hydroxyapatite) (Klevezal 1996). Enamel is formed completely before tooth eruption (Klevezal 1996).

Dentine forms the majority of the substance of the tooth and is very tough and resilient (Hillson 1986). It is a mineralized tubular tissue composed of cells, together with an intercellular substance. The crown dentine is covered with enamel, and the root dentine is covered with cementum. Dentine is less hard than enamel, but harder than bone and cementum. It has a higher organic component than enamel (Scott and Symons 1974).

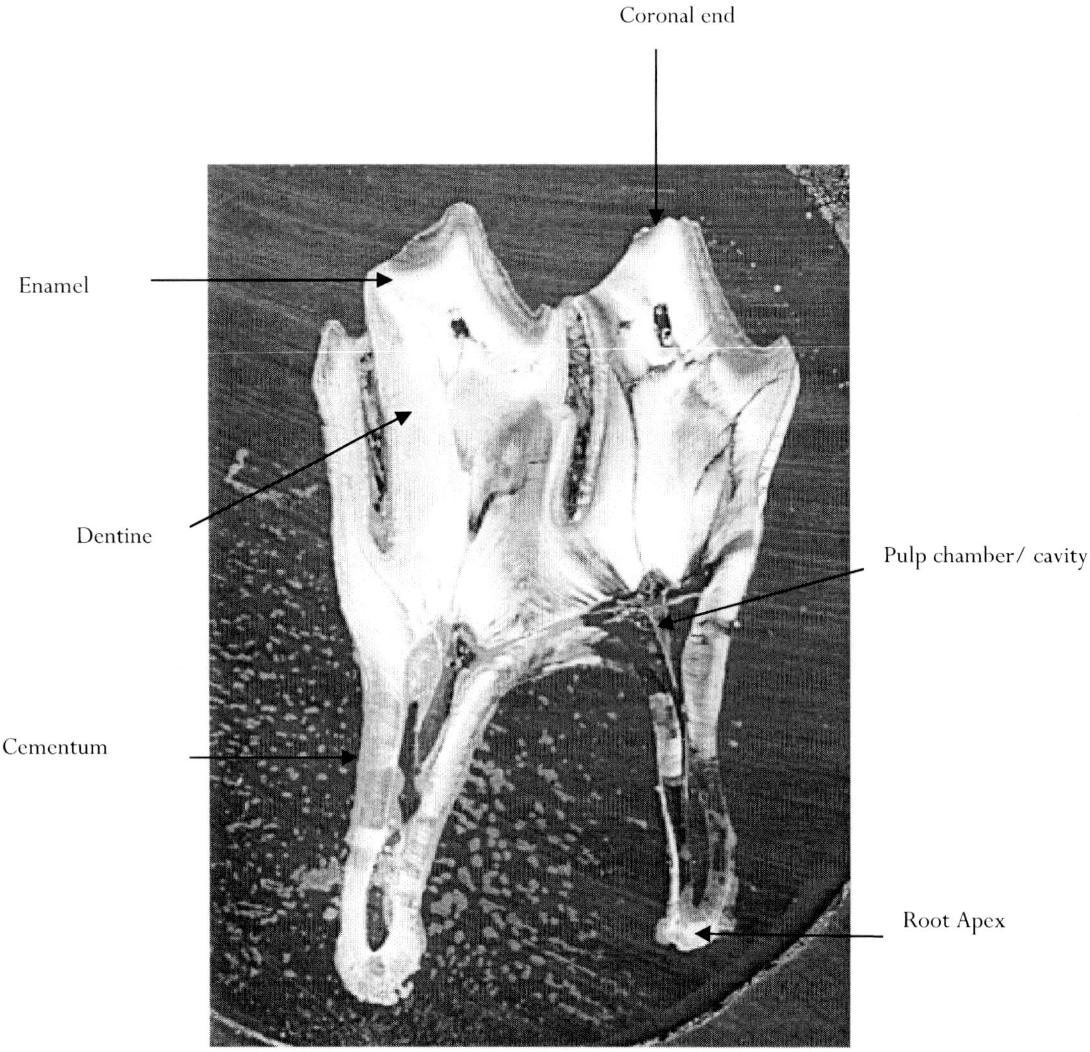

The **Pulp Chamber** is the area in the middle of the root from the base to the tip, surrounded by the dentine of the crown and root. The pulp within this chamber is a soft cellular tissue which supplies the nerves and blood to the tooth (Hillson 1986). The pulp contains soft tissues which provide for nutrition and growth of the tooth (Klevezal 1996).

Cementum normally covers the entire root, overlaying and being firmly adhered to the dentine in a thin layer. It is composed of an organic matrix and an inorganic element. Its main function is to anchor the tooth into the surrounding bone via the periodontal ligament which is an integral part of the cementum. In horse, sheep, goat, and cattle cementum may also cover part of the crown.

All teeth are structured in this way, although they vary in height, width, the number of folds in the enamel, and of extra mounds in the enamel known as cusps (Hillson 1986).The tooth is held into the jaw in a socket called the alveolar bone. Collagen fibres of the periodontal ligament hold the tooth into this socket: they are attached both to the tooth and to the surrounding bone. They also allow the tooth to move through the bone in response to wear. It is because of the flexibility of the collagen fibres and the cells of the periodontal ligament that teeth are able to erupt into their functional position. The ligament also enables the tooth to move in response to wear.

A number of terms are commonly used by researchers in cementum incremental analysis to describe areas of observation of cementum layering. These can be found in Appendix 1.

Figure 2. First Molar of a Red deer in the jaw

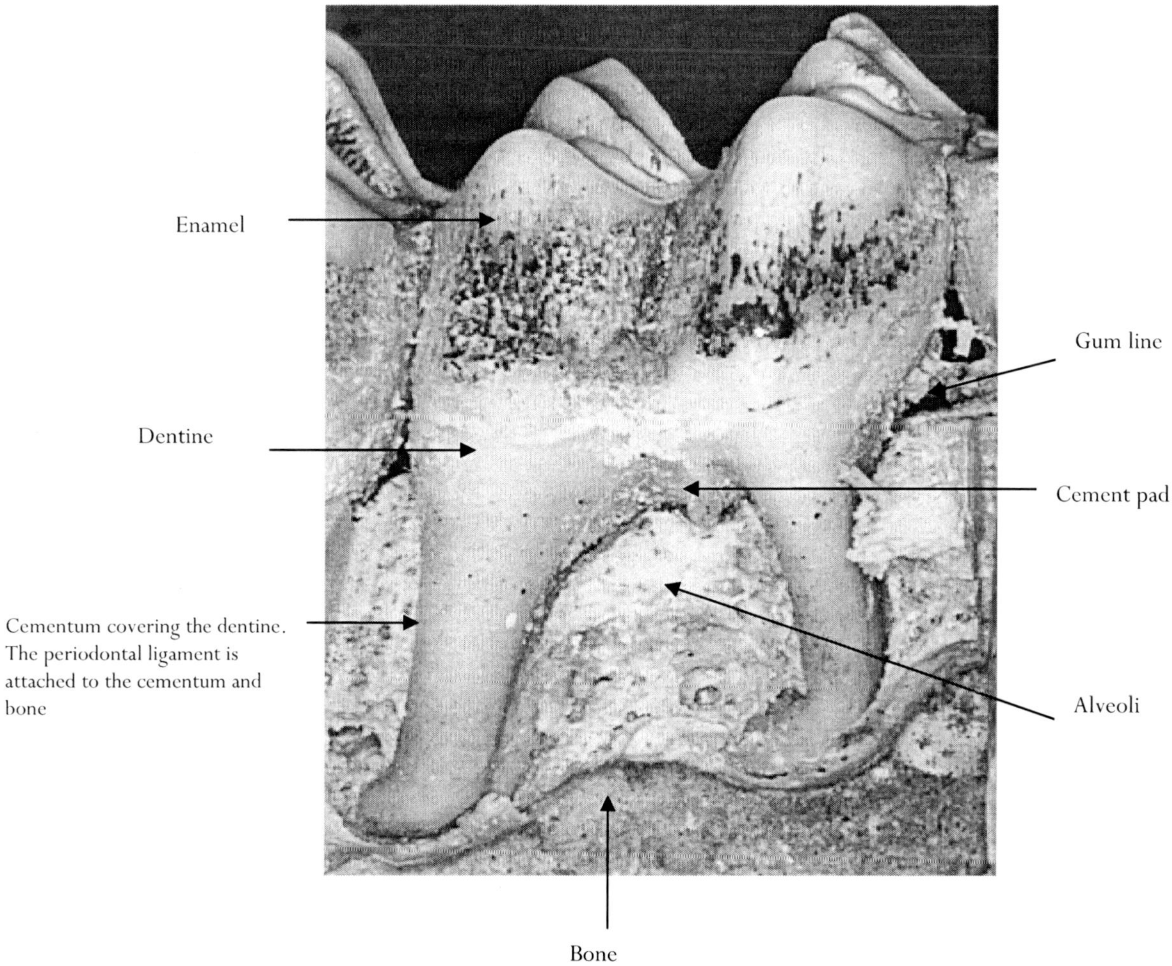

2. DISTRIBUTION, FUNCTION, AND COMPOSITION OF CEMENTUM

Cementum is a pale yellow substance with a dull surface. It is less yellow than dentine and is also less hard (Henderson Scott 1982). In most mammals, including Red deer and man, it extends from the cementum-enamel junction to cover the dentine of the root; in some other mammals, it can also be present on the crown. For example, the entire crown and infundibulum are covered with cementum in the cow and the horse (Hillson 1986), and substantial deposits have been found on the enamel of sperm whale (Klevezal 1996). It varies substantially in thickness at different levels of the root, being thickest at the apex and in the inter radicular areas (that is, the areas between the roots of multi-rooted teeth, sometimes also called the pad) (typically 50-200μm), and thinnest cervically (typically 10-50 μm) (Berkovitz 1995).

The function of cementum

Most authors agree that cementum has a number of functions. The first is to anchor the tooth into its socket by attachment of the periodontal ligament to the tooth surface: the fibres of the periodontal ligament are embedded into the cementum, thereby attaching the tooth to the alveolar bone (Scott & Symons 1974). The formation of cementum continues throughout life and the attachment of the periodontal fibres can be altered or shifted according to the functional needs of the tooth; moreover, newly formed periodontal fibres can gain attachment to the tooth, replacing fibres which have aged. This necessity for a shifting of periodontal fibres is most obvious in the vertical movement of the teeth during their eruption, but is equally important to allow the bodily lateral and mesial movement of the teeth in the jaws during their growth and the mesial movements which occur afterwards as a result of occlusal wear. As well as the very marked movements of the teeth, continual minute adjustments for each tooth occur in response to changing pressure applied when the teeth are in use (Henderson Scott 1982). Thus a major function seems to be to compensate for tooth movement due to wear on the occlusal surfaces: cementum is responsible for adding length to the tooth to ensure that the tooth remains at a level of use within the mouth as it is continually worn down on the occlusal plane, as well as for compensating for movement within the jaw, including eruption. Teeth must erupt as they wear down in order to maintain a consistent inter-occlusal surface between maxillary and mandibular teeth (Brown and Chapman 1990). In contrast to this, it may be that cementum is laid down to fill the gap left between the bone and the tooth root once the tooth has moved up to bring the enamel into wear, thereby reacting to, rather than causing the eruption (Brown 1997 pers. comm.). Other theories have also been advanced within this broad framework: for example, Jones (in Osborn 1981) suggests that cementum contributes to the size and strength of the root, and protects the encased dentine of the root.

According to Bosshardt and Selvig (1997), "the dynamic and highly responsive features of cementum are crucial for maintaining occlusal relationship and for the integrity of the root surface and its function in tooth support". Thus teeth are undergoing constant change throughout life, as the tooth responds to changing functional demands by selective apposition, resorption, and repair of cementum (Osborn 1981). This statement is in stark contrast to the claims of some archaeologists and other researchers in the field of incremental analysis, who claim that, once laid down, cementum is rarely resorbed (Lieberman 1993, Lieberman and Meadow 1992). It is clear that some experience is required to identify these life changes in cementum deposition, and that it is unrealistic to expect to interpret cementum layering before a thorough understanding of cementum formation has been attained (Lieberman and Meadow 1992).

Cementum is softer and more permeable than dentine, and its surface cells remain active and able to create or remove cementum (Osborn 1981) until the cementum covered root erupts into the mouth. Up to that stage, it is the most adaptable member of the periodontum, and is continually modified to accommodate changes due to both external and internal factors. Once out of the peridontium it can no longer be altered, or repaired. Another consequence of its softness is that, as the tooth erupts and brings cementum into the mouth, the exposed cementum is subject to relatively rapid wear. The implication of this for incremental analysis is that, once the tooth has erupted, the cementum-enamel junction is no longer a suitable location for the study of incremental layers since cementum is subject to wear once it is above the gum line. Archaeologists often note that one of the benefits of cementum incremental analysis is that it can be used on isolated teeth (Pike-Tay 1991, Gordon 1988, Beasley 1987). If isolated teeth are used, there is no secure way of ensuring that the cementum was all below the gum line, or protected throughout life. This point should be emphasized, since the cementum-enamel junction is often cited as the best area for cementum incremental studies, due to the ease with which increments can be identified there.

The composition of cementum

The overall chemical composition of cementum is similar to bone (Jones in Osborn 1981). By weight, cementum consists of approximately 65% inorganic material, 23% organic material, and 12% water (Berkovitz et al 1995). The principal inorganic component is an impure form of hydroxyapatite (Calcium Phosphate), while the organic matrix is primarily collagen and ground substance. Ground substance is an amorphous, organic material containing proteoglycans (Hillson 1986). The collagen is similar to that found in bone and is discussed in more detail below.

Cementum is formed on the surface of dentine and enamel by cementoblasts, which are cubic cells forming a single layer in contact with the dentine (Scott & Symons 1974). Cementogenesis, the process of cementum formation and its subsequent mineralisation, is complex and not fully understood - it will be discussed in more detail once the different types of cementum have been described. The composition of cementum varies even within a single tooth, and since the change in composition is continuous, any classification scheme is necessarily somewhat arbitrary. There are however two distinct methods of classification which are commonly used, one of which is based upon the presence or absence of cells, and the other upon the nature and origin of the collagen fibres which make up the organic matrix. Before embarking on a discussion of these two schemes, it should be noted that there are two exceptional types of cementum which must be distinguished from the remainder. First, there is *intermediate cementum*, which forms a thin layer between the granular layer of Tomes[1] and the main bulk of the cementum. It is typically deposited before the tooth has fully erupted and has come into occlusion (Lieberman & Meadow 1992). It is the only form of cementum which is *afibrillar* (i.e. contains no collagen fibres), and as such the classification based upon the origin of collagen fibres is not applicable to it. However the existence of this intermediate cementum is disputed in some species: thus for example, Bosshardt and Selvig (1997) write "The term intermediate cementum appears repeatedly in the literature and in textbooks. Although originally described for the apical portion of human teeth, there exists no interfacial layer between dentine and cementum in human teeth. In rodent molars and incisors on the other hand, an intermediate layer has frequently been observed, particularly between acellular extrinsic fibre cementum and dentine." As noted earlier, the possibility of an intermediate layer would add confusion or likely misinterpretation of the cementum layers if the observer were inexperienced. Second, there is *cementoid* or *precementum*, a thin layer of unmineralized cementum, lined by cementoblasts, which

[1]The granular layer of Tomes is a layer of dentine that is granular in appearance and is located immediately beneath the cement.

borders the mineralized cementum where the matrix is being deposited. In growing cementum a layer of precement covers the surface (Hillson 1986). Lieberman and Meadow (1992) identify that precementum isn't present on all parts of the tooth root, but it is important in the development of cementum as it seems to regulate the variations in the nature of the cementum that is deposited. They also note that research on this layer of incompletely calcified tissue will be critical in determining which factors regulate cementogenesis (after Rose et al 1987, McAlister et al 1990), particularly those which result in layering. The existence and nature of precementum should also be taken into consideration when performing incremental analysis on archaeological teeth, since the cementum which is in formation is unlikely to survive in the ground, and may therefore contribute to error in the analysis.

Acellular and cellular (primary and secondary) cementum

The first classification is based simply upon the presence or absence of cells within the cementum: cellular cementum contains cells (cementocytes) which are entrapped cementoblasts, whereas acellular cementum does not. The alternative terms primary (acellular) and secondary (cellular) are sometimes used, on the grounds that acellular cementum is formed before cellular. Acellular cementum is distributed towards the crown, though typically acellular cementum covers the root of the tooth, adjacent to the dentine, from the cementum-enamel junction to the neighbourhood of the apex: it may cover the entire root of incisors or canines (Scott & Symons 1974). Acellular cementum is formed at a slow rate and cementoblasts remain on the surface of the cementum and do not become embedded in the tissue (Hillson 1986). Cellular cementum, on the other hand, is formed in the apical area, in the interradicular area of multi-rooted teeth, or on top of the acellular. It is extremely scarce, and may be entirely absent, in human anterior teeth (Scott & Symons 1974). There are, however frequent exceptions to this typical distribution. Cellular cementum is rapidly deposited and is less mineralized than acellular cementum (Hillson 1986). Acellular cementum may be formed on top of cellular cementum, and several layers of the two types may alternate in an apparently random manner (Ten Cate 1989). "In some areas, the two variants of cementum alternate irregularly, probably representing variations in the rate of deposition" (Berkovitz et al 1995). This is another important point in incremental analysis, since without the ability to distinguish between the different types of cementum, one could easily confuse the alternation of cementum layers with the alternation of cellular and acellular cementum, and therefore misinterpret both age and season of death. As Berkovitz et al (1995) note, "in acellular cementum, incremental lines tend to be close together, thin and even. In the more rapidly formed cellular cementum, incremental lines are further apart, thicker and more irregular."

One of the most important differences between the two types of cementum is that cellular cementum is formed much more quickly than the acellular variety. Indeed, the greater rate of formation is thought to be responsible for the presence of cells in cellular cementum: in acellular cementum the forming cementoblasts retreat, leaving the cementum matrix behind, whereas in cellular cementum the cementoblasts become trapped in lacunae within their own matrix, and become embedded in the tissue as cementocytes. The wider precementum layer and the more widely spaced incremental layers in cellular cementum are also accounted for by the increased rate of formation (Berkovitz et al 1995).

The following table (after Berkovitz et al 1995) summarizes the main differences between acellular and cellular cementum:

Acellular	Cellular
No cells	Lacunae and canaliculi containing cementocytes and their processes
Rate of development relatively slow	Rate of development relatively fast
Border with dentine not clearly demarcated	Border with dentine clearly demarcated
Incremental lines relatively close together	Incremental lines relatively wide apart
Precementum layer narrow	Precementum layer wide

Table 1: Difference between cellular and acellular cementum.

Extrinsic fibre, mixed fibre, and intrinsic fibre cementum

The organic matrix of cementum has two sources. First, there are fibres formed outside the cementum by the fibroblasts of the periodontal ligament that have become incorporated into the cementum. These are called *extrinsic fibres*, or *Sharpey's fibres,* and continue into the cementum in the same direction as the fibres of the ligament: that is, approximately perpendicular to the root surface. Second, there are fibres formed by the cementoblasts (cementum forming cells), which are called *intrinsic fibres*. These run parallel to the root surface. Cementum (with the exception of afibrillar intermediate cementum) can therefore be classified according as the collagen fibres which make up its organic matrix are extrinsic, intrinsic, or a mixture of the two. Extrinsic fibre cementum is always acellular, and intrinsic fibre cementum always cellular. Mixed fibre cementum may be cellular or acellular, depending on the rate of formation.

Cementogenesis

The process of cementum formation and mineralisation will be discussed following the treatment of Berkovitz et al. (1995), considering first the formation of primary and then of secondary cementum. It should be emphasized that this process is not well understood at present, and the mechanisms outlined here are for the most part unconfirmed.

Primary (acellular) cementum
As has already been mentioned, much of the collagen in acellular cementum is derived from Sharpey's fibres of the periodontal ligament. The cementoblasts therefore secrete little collagen, although they are assumed to secrete components of ground substance: this assumption is supported by the presence within cementoblasts of the components necessary for protein synthesis. However, the fact that the cementoblasts are only contributing ground substance, taken in conjunction with the slow rate of formation of acellular cementum, implies that the cementoblasts involved in primary cementum production do not have the cytological features of highly productive cells. Once laid down as precementum or cementoid, the mineralisation of the newly formed cementum layer does not appear to be controlled by the cells, whose role is probably limited to providing the medium in which mineralisation occurs, rather than the mineral ions themselves. It is likely, instead, that mineralisation is induced by the presence of hydroxyapatite in the neighboring dentine.

Secondary (cellular) cementum
Following the formation of primary cementum in the cervical portion of the root, secondary cementum is created in the apical region at about the time of eruption. The cementoblasts responsible for the production of cellular cementum secrete intrinsic collagen fibres as well as ground substance. This, coupled with the greater rate of formation of secondary cementum, explains the presence in the cementoblasts of cytological features associated with highly productive cells. The orientation and arrangement of the intrinsic fibres is thought to be due to the movement of the cells with respect to the surface which they are forming. The precement layer is much more evident in secondary cementum, reaching a thickness of 5μm in man.

The mineralisation of secondary cementum appears to take place independently in the extrinsic fibres, intrinsic fibres, and ground substance. It takes place preferentially along the length of the fibres: hence the directions of mineralisation along the extrinsic and intrinsic fibres are perpendicular to each other. The extrinsic fibres are much thicker than the intrinsic, and accordingly mineralize much more slowly. Thus the mineral surface of mixed fibre secondary cementum is marked with holes corresponding to the extrinsic fibres. Mineralisation of the ground substance takes place after that of the fibres.

In general, the more rapidly cementum is formed, the less highly mineralized it will be. Thus cellular cementum is usually less well mineralized than acellular.

3. INCREMENTAL LAYERS IN CEMENTUM

Roughly speaking, cementum is composed of alternating layers: thicker layers, which are translucent and hence appear light under transmitted light, and thinner layers, which are opaque, and hence appear dark under transmitted light. The terms "dark" and "light" layers are unsuitable, since translucent layers appear dark and opaque layers appear light when viewed under reflected light. The appearance of the layers also depends upon the type of section being studied - one of the major difficulties in this area is that there is frequent confusion in the literature as to which type of section and which type of microscope is being used: at times, the terminology is confused even within the scope of a single paper. The layers range in thickness between 10 and 130 microns (Omar 1992, Lieberman and Meadow 1992).

It is generally assumed that the deposition of cementum in many mammals which leads to incremental layers approximately follows an annual cycle (Hillson 1986). It is furthermore commonly accepted that the thicker translucent layer is formed during the summer, and that the thinner opaque layer is formed during the winter. For this reason, the opaque layers are often referred to as "restlines", implying a period of slower growth. However, since neither the nature nor the causes of the incremental structure are well understood, as will be made clear below, this terminology should also be resisted. Berkovitz et al (1996) summed up this point: "cementum is deposited in an irregular rhythm, resulting in unevenly spaced incremental lines. Unlike enamel and dentine, the precise periodicity between the incremental lines is unknown, although there have been unsuccessful attempts to relate it to the annual cycle."

The basic assumption behind cementum incremental analysis (see Klevezal and Kleinberg 1967, Morris 1972, Casteel 1976, Stallibrass 1982 and Gordon 1991, Klevezal 1996 for surveys covering a wide range of species) is that, since one translucent and one opaque layer are laid down in each year, the age of an animal can be estimated by counting the number of translucent-opaque pairs (and adding to this the age of eruption of the tooth). Moreover, it should be possible to estimate the season of death of an animal by determining whether the outermost layer is translucent (summer death) or opaque (winter death). It is also assumed that greater accuracy can be obtained by comparing the width of the outermost layer to an estimate of the width which it would have had, had it been completed. A study of possible methods for performing such calculations is presented in Monks and Johnston (1993). Aitken (1975) studied a collection of 74 Roe deer jaws (9 of known age), and found that for animals shot in autumn (August 3rd to December 5th) there was a white band comprised of cementocytes, and that for those shot in winter (January) there was a thin line of dark acellular material. Of those shot between these periods, the outermost layer was composed of dark cellular cementum in 60% of the animals, and contained abundant cementocytes in the other 40%.

Almost all authors agree that the situation is much more complicated than is suggested by this description, that considerable skill is required on the part of the observer, and that accurate results cannot be guaranteed. One of the main contentions of this study is that, in fact, the complications and difficulties are sufficiently great that it is not possible to obtain fully accurate information by means of cementum incremental analysis using standard ground thin sections.

4. PROBLEMS OF TERMINOLOGY

It has been recognized that inconsistent terminology in the literature has compounded problems of the interpretation of cementum increments (Burke 1995, Gordon 1991, Pike-Tay 1991, Lieberman 1992). In choosing and defining terms with which to describe incremental structures, there are two pitfalls that it is important to avoid. First, it can be misleading to make use of optical properties that depend upon a particular type of microscopy: for example, regions which appear dark under polarized transmitted light will appear light when viewed under reflected light. Second, because the nature, causes, and seasonality of incremental structures have not been conclusively established (as described later in this chapter), theory-laden terms such as 'summer', 'winter', 'active', and 'rest' should also be avoided. A number of different schemes have been proposed by various authors, some of which will be described shortly. The terminology used in this study is as follows: the incremental structure is composed of **bands** and **lines**, distinguished by the fact that bands appear lighter, or whiter, than lines when viewed under **polarized transmitted light**. When it is necessary to refer to bands and lines indiscriminately, the term **layers** is used: a layer is either a band or a line. Bands are generally, but not always, wider than lines, and are often associated with a period of more rapid growth, and hence also with the summer; while lines are often associated with a period of 'rest' or arrested growth, and hence with the winter.

The relationship with terminology proposed by some other authors is summarized below:

- **Burke and Castanet (1995):** "*Growth layers* will refer to any layering in dental cementum or bone which is the result of appositional (sometimes termed incremental) growth. The term *growth zones* will designate the relatively thick, opaque layers of "summer" or active cementum growth which are isotropic. *Annuli* refers to the narrower, anisotropic bands of relatively translucent cementum or bone. The annuli correspond to periods of slow growth. *Lines of arrested growth* (LAGs) designate thin, chromophile discontinuities, or "rest lines", in cementum, sometimes situated within annuli (when these latter are present), sometimes alternating with growth zones when annuli are absent. LAGs, which correspond to the "adhesion lines" of Klevezal and Kleinberg (1967) and the "incremental growth lines" of Grue and Jensen (1979), represent "inundated surface regions". LAGs appear bright under ordinary transmitted light, and highly birefringent under polarized light. Annuli and LAGs correspond to periods of slowed and arrested tissue growth respectively." As an explanatory footnote, they add that "An opaque body (e.g. growth zones in cement) will appear bright (white) under reflected natural light, and dark (black) under transmitted natural light. A translucent body (e.g. annuli in cement) will have inverse properties, appearing dark under reflected natural light, and bright under transmitted light". Thus the zones of Burke and Castanet correspond to bands, and the annuli and LAGs to lines. There appears to be an error in these definitions, since bands are in fact translucent, while lines are opaque. Notice that the term "Lines of arrested growth" is theory-laden. The terms "zones" and "annuli" appear to be arbitrary: no reason is given why zones should not be called annuli and vice-versa.

- **Lieberman (1994)** refers simply to *opaque bands* and *translucent bands*, stressing that these terms refer to the appearance of the layers when viewed under transmitted cross-polarized light, and that the optical nature of cementum depends on the orientation of the collagen relative to that of the polarizers, so that a fixed orientation should be used.
- **Gordon (1984)** is a paper dedicated to discussing the problems of terminology in incremental analysis. After summarizing a number of possible systems, he adopts the terms *translucent increment* and *opaque increment*, explaining that "A translucent increment is light in transmitted light and stain, dark in reflected light because it absorbs light and stain, and is the ridge in etched teeth. An opaque increment is dark in transmitted light and stain, light in reflected light because it reflects light, and forms the grooves in etched teeth."
- **Pike-Tay (1991)** adopts a variety of terms, including *band*, *layer*, *annulus*, and *line*, generally making the distinction between translucent and opaque structures. She agrees with the need for standardization of terminology expressed in Gordon (1984).

5. CAUSES OF CEMENTUM LAYERING

It is assumed that the deposition of cementum occurs rhythmically, with periods of activity alternating with periods of quiescence. The periods of slower growth are associated with growth layers which are believed to have a higher content of ground substance and mineral compared to the adjacent cementum (Berkovitz et al 1995). Though the layers may be explained in this way, very little is known about the cause of this layering and there are differences of opinion as to whether or not the increments truly reflect seasons, or even (in some cases) years, in the life of an animal. In this section I shall discuss: first, the nature of growth layers (that is, the biological structures which give rise to alternating bands and lines); secondly, some theories of the biological origin of the layers (which external and internal stimuli induce layering, and whether or not these stimuli may account for the seasonal nature of the layers); third, some of the various problems which different authors have encountered in their attempts to age animals using incremental analysis (without, in this chapter, entering into the question of sectioning technique, which will be treated in detail in Chapter 3); and finally, the necessity of studying a large known-aged sample before attempting any analysis of specimens of unknown age. Berkovitz et al (1995) note that "the appearance of incremental lines in cementum is mainly due to differences in the degree of mineralisation, but these must also reflect differences in composition of the underlying matrix since the lines are readily visible in decalcified sections." This suggests that different sectioning techniques will provide different information. It should also be noted that there may be variations in cementum deposition between species, and very little work has been attempted that crosses different species from the same environment. This should be taken into consideration in this study, which is based on the study of one species only. In a later chapter, I shall present a systematic study of growth layers at a number of different locations on the teeth of a large known-aged sample of red deer, in order to demonstrate that, for this species at least, it is not even possible to obtain an accurate age using incremental analysis, let alone information about the season of death.

The nature of cementum increments

The differences in composition of bands and lines in cementum are not well understood, and indeed little research has been devoted to this problem (Selvig 1965, Boyde and Jones 1972, Jones 1987). Although it is assumed that the pattern of layers can be attributed to different densities, there is speculation as to why this should be and what are the constituents of the different densities. Amongst the many conjectures made are:

1. That the lines are hypercalcified (Klevezal and Kleinberg 1967). This assumes that there is more calcium in the lines than there are in the bands. This is agreed by Kubota et al (1963), Ohsumi et al (1963).

2. That the bands are hypercalcified (McLaren 1958, Sergeant 1959, 1962, Berzin 1961, 1964).

3. That the different optical properties arise from a variation in density due to different mineralization rates (Jones 1981, Davis 1986, Klevezal and Kleinberg 1967, Boyde and Jones 1972, Hillson 1986). Boyde and Jones associate the mineralization pattern with the relative proportions of extrinsic and intrinsic fibres, in turn related to the speed of tissue deposition. The rate at which cementum is formed depends upon the activity of the cementoblasts. When the rate is slow and the intrinsic fibre component is small the incremental layers are even and thin so no cells are incorporated. As the proportion of intrinsic fibres rises the thickness of the cementum layer increases more rapidly and the incremental layers, and hence the cementum surface, are less regular. A rapid production of intrinsic matrix and consequent embedding of extrinsic fibres also leads to the incorporation of cells within the cementum. The increments in cellular cementum are generally patchy and uneven and the incremental layers are more widely spaced: the plane of the root surface is parallel with the plane of the dentine-cementum junction. As the rate of production slows, the number of cementoblasts trapped in the tissue is reduced and the cementum may become acellular. Layers of acellular and cellular cementum may alternate on a root surface, indicating variation in the appositional rate. The thickness of the unmineralized matrix, the precement (or cementoid) at the surface also varies with the appositional rate and is greatest during cellular cementum formation. The rate and amount of cellular cementum deposition is probably related to the degree of eruption, the amount of wear in a given tooth, and the overall size of the tooth.

4. That the differences, in acellular cementum, are due to differences in the orientation of Sharpey's fibres (Lieberman 1993, 1994). Hydroxyapatite crystals in cementum are precipitated along a pre-existing collagen matrix (Lowenstam and Weiner 1989 after Lieberman 1992), so that changes in the orientation of the collagen fibre bundles will affect the optical behavior of different layers. The angle of collagen bundles in acellular cementum changes between layers, Sharpey's fibres probably responding to extrinsic forces exerted on the tooth during occlusion, resulting in a more acute angle relative to the orientation of the mineralizing front under greater occlusal forces. Under this conjecture, the layers would arise as a consequence of seasonal variations in the biomechanical stresses placed on teeth.

The causes of cementum increments

There is no general agreement on the nature of the external and internal stimuli which induce cementum layering. Early researchers suggested that incremental layers were the result of extremes of climate or lifestyle causing massive metabolic changes (Stott et al 1982). More recently, researchers have come to the conclusion that causal factors are complicated and cannot be isolated (Pike-Tay 1991). It is assumed, however, that some elements are constant, such as the fact that cementum layers are deposited throughout life and that the thicker layers represent a period of growth. (Pike-Tay 1991). Pike-Tay goes further with this assumption and claims that the period of growth can be roughly associated with "summer" and the season of arrested growth with "winter". I prefer to leave this as a possibility rather than an assumption until further research is undertaken on large modern populations of known age and season of death. Ideally animals should be studied using annual detectable dyes, as without a clear discriminating marker it will not be possible to say if the lines or bands are associated with seasons (Brown pers. comm.1999). A number of factors have been proposed as possible causes of the annual cycle of cementum deposition: amongst the most important are:

- Nutrition: the quality and quantity of food available to the animal. Seasonal contrasts in diet (McEwan, Low and Cowan 1963, Klevezal and Kleinberg 1967, Hillson 1986, Gordon 1988).

- Biomechanical changes: for example, the stress to which teeth are subjected (Saxon and Higham 1968, Lieberman and Meadow 1992).
- Hormonal changes with the regression and development of sexual organs, moult, antler growth and antler casting (Klevezal and Kleinberg 1967, Kolb 1978).
- Climatic changes.
- Changes in the metabolic rate or physiology (Grue 1976, Hillson 1986).

One explanation for the difficulty of distinguishing between these factors is that the incremental structure may be well correlated with "basic events in an animal's life" (Klevezal 1970), but these basic events may impact upon several of the potential causal factors. For example, it is claimed that the teeth of red deer stags undergo a transition from band to a line during the rut (Mitchell 1967). However, this transition could be due to nutritional changes (the stags have a much reduced food intake during the rut), to biomechanical changes (the teeth are under much reduced stress because of the reduced food intake: mechanical stress must have some effect on the underlying cementum, if it is the case that cementum is formed to keep the tooth in wear and anchored to the periodontium), or to hormonal changes. Moreover, it is not always straightforward to associate the incremental structure with such basic life events with any degree of confidence: there are substantial variations in the observed incremental structure both between species and within given species. Similarly, Saxon and Higham (1968) observed that decreased food availability in winter results in reduced tooth wear in herbivores, with an associated decrease in the rate of cementum formation. However, other factors such as the hardness of the food and its nutritional content also need to be considered. Mitchell (1963, 1967) considers that the annual pattern of cementum deposition is more closely related to body growth and condition than with any other features of the annual cycle. He states that, although the rate of eruption of each tooth never completely compensates for crown wear, the two are nevertheless clearly related: for example, molar teeth have thicker deposits of cementum than incisors or canines, and teeth which show abnormal wear have correspondingly thicker deposits. This variation also has obvious consequences for the accuracy of incremental analysis, particularly when the widths of increments are used to establish seasonality (Burke 1991), or when isolated teeth are being studied, when it may not be clear that a tooth is abnormally worn.

I believe that a number of the factors which have been proposed can be discounted by means of the simple observation that cementum increments are discrete rather than continuous, and must therefore be caused by discrete rather than continuous phenomena. For instance, if the main causal factor were nutrition, then one would expect a gradual change in the optical properties of the cementum throughout the year as food supplies gradually increased or decreased, rather than the discrete changes which are in fact observed.

A number of authors have carried out experiments or made observations in an attempt to isolate the causes of cementum layering, without, however, reaching any consensus.

- Lieberman (1993) experimented with the diets of six goats that were kept for 12 months under identical conditions with the exception of their diet. Two goats were fed throughout the 12 months on the same diet, two were fed the same diet but for four months the diet was softened, and the last two were fed food of the same hardness as the first two, but with reduced protein, vitamins and minerals for four months. For the four months of changing diet the tissue deposited was labelled with fluorochrome dyes (oxytetracyline, calcein, and alizarin). Lieberman concluded that the Sharpey's fibres change as a response to the hardness of the food, rather than the nutritional content, and that therefore cementum bands preserve seasonal variations in Sharpey's fibre orientation. Though his results may have demonstrated that Sharpey's fibres alter with the degree of hardness of the food being consumed, there is some difficulty in associating this directly with seasonal changes in the hardness of food consumption for many mammals that demonstrate incremental layering, such as carnivores (Grue 1976, Kolb 1978).
- Gordon (1988) specifically suggests that the lines are darker due to a higher calcium phosphate content: this arises because blood calcium level is constant throughout the year, whereas protein intake is reduced during the winter. Under this theory, lines correspond to periods of reduced protein availability.
- Grue (1976) observed that mink reduce their food intake during the winter, even when they are raised on farms and are fed a steady diet. The choice to reduce food intake suggests a change in metabolic rate, which could be the actual stimulus responsible for layering.
- Mundy and Fuller (1964) found that cementum increments are much easier to read in Grizzly bears than in either Caribou (Rangifer Tarandus) or Bison (Bison bison). They attribute the difference to the "sharp contrast between summer and winter and to the alternating periods of use and disuse of the teeth". This observation could support nutrition, biomechanical changes, climatic changes, or changes in metabolic rate as underlying causes of layering. To complete the picture, they also note that the rate of deposition of cementum changes with age, the first five annuli being wider and clearer than those deposited after the age of five. They suggest that this may be related to the onset of sexual maturity, thus associating hormonal changes with incremental structure. Kolb (1978) also suggests a connection with the reproductive cycle: studying the premolars of unknown age foxes from Scotland, he found that there were significant differences between sexes in each area, but not between areas within a given sex. Aitken (1975) observed no differences between Roe deer from Dorset: one of a sample of five known aged

animals was a three year old castrate captive buck which showed two thick white bands and the beginnings of a third; this was almost identical to a four year old wild animal from the same area. This would seem to suggest that nutrition has little to do with cementum deposition. The only notable difference was the presence of darker bands within the white ones in the wild animal, which Aitken attributes to the rut.

- Other authors have claimed that, for certain species, geographical location does affect the incremental structure. Roberts (1978), studying coyote, observed that there is "considerable variation in the degree of clarity and definition of annuli in specimens collected from different geographic areas". Allen and Kohn (1976) also found marked differences between known aged coyotes from different locations. They conclude that cementum incremental analysis is not a reliable method of ageing, since the precise timing of cementum formation cannot be established. Aitken (1975) studied two known aged populations of Roe deer, one from Cheddington and one from Thetford, and found that there was a marked difference in the pattern of cementum deposition between the two populations. He noted that while the Thetford deer showed clearly defined bands of even thickness, the Cheddington deer showed poorly defined bands, often incomplete and variable in number and separated by minimal amounts of acellular cementum. He attributes this to the difference that the climate has on food availability and differences in genetics. Stoneberg and Jonkel (1966), studying Brown bear, also urged caution. They found that the "winter line" in Brown bear is produced prior to hibernation, and concluded that although layering seems to correlate with age and seasonality, the causes are not understood and further investigation is needed. Within a given species, populations in areas with more continental climates generally have a clearer and more definite layering pattern than those from oceanic climates (Leader-Williams 1979). There may therefore be many animals in which distinct cementum increments cannot be detected.
- Miller (1974) measured tooth wear on Caribou, and noted that males show more wear than females, with mean wear for 7 year old males being comparable to that of 8 year old females. He proposes that this is because the male needs to eat more to maintain body weight. If this is the case, then further research is needed to establish whether or not cementum is deposited differently in male and female animals. One might suppose that layers would be thicker in males if they are subject to more rapid wear.
- Secondary and false increments, discussed in more detail below, have also added to the debate on the causes of cementum layering.

Though it is acknowledged that the causes of incremental bands are not well understood, many researchers do not believe that this is a problem. Landon (1993) in his study of cattle, pig and caprid teeth sums this up by claiming "this does not, however, negate the validity of the technique, even though the causation is not completely understood, the seasonal incrementation pattern of tooth cementum has been recognised in a wide variety of different mammals".

6. PROBLEMS WITH INCREMENTAL ANALYSIS

A number of authors have expressed unease about the accuracy and reliability of the estimation of age or season of death using cementum incremental analysis. Some attribute this to misunderstandings by other researchers and others to more substantial obstacles, which may or may not be surmountable. Thus, for example, Grau et al. (1970) write that "the inaccuracy of the technique might be due to cementum layers which do not form annually, variations in histological technique, inability to differentiate and count closer layers in older specimens, or to a combination of these and other factors. The artificial environment and non-varying diet of captive animals may affect the formation of layers, but it seems pointless to speculate on this until more is known about the formation of the layers". Lieberman and Meadow (1992), on the other hand, explain the problems in attempting to use cellular cementum for incremental analysis: "it is crucial to recognize that while the growth of cellular cementum is generally phasic because of the long periods of cementoblast activity, there is currently limited evidence that these growth periods are strongly seasonal. Rest layers in cellular cementum could therefore result from different lengths of time. This means that while cellular cementum increments may yield information about an individual's age of death, they are not always useful for estimating season of death". Matson, in his 1989 Progress Report no. 11, lists four common misunderstandings about ageing by means of cementum:

1. That dark cementum bands are caused by environmental factors.
2. That teeth of mammals from southern regions lack distinct cementum layers because of the mild winters.
3. That the cementum ageing method will always produce precisely correct results, and
4. That any tooth type can be used to determine the age of any species.

He claims that "there is no evidence that points to any physiological or environmental factor as an important influence upon cyclic cementum growth".

Gasaway, Harkness and Rausch (1978), studying moose, demonstrate using known aged specimens that there are great variations in the ageing of animals by means of cementum, and that there are also differences between different observers (this point will be considered in detail in Chapter 4). They do, however, note that there does appear to be definite layering correlating with seasons. Moore et al. (1995), comparing five different techniques for estimating the age of a sample of 27 Fallow deer of known age, found cementum analysis to be unsatisfactory, only providing an accurate age in 53% of the animals. The accuracy could arguably have been affected by their technique, however: they examined thick cut sections under a binocular microscope. They found a tendency for cementum analysis to underestimate the true age although, in contrast with other researchers working on different species (see below), they did not find the method more inaccurate for older animals. Brown and Chapman (1990) also state that cementum incremental analysis is inaccurate for the population of Fallow deer which they studied. Roberts (1978), studying layering in coyote, found that the number of layers varies between different teeth of the same animal, and that they tend to merge together in incisors making them difficult to distinguish.

The difficulties experienced with cementum incremental analysis are even more acute when older animals are considered. Many researchers have found that accuracy is severely impaired at the top of the age range, with the point at which this begins to occur being species-dependent. For example, Grau et al. (1970) found that in raccoons, the technique can only be relied upon for animals aged up to 60 months. Craighead, Craighead and McCutchen (1970) also note the difficulty of distinguishing separate layers in older Grizzly bears. Turner (1977) observed that the amount of cementum laid down in North American sheep decreases with age and there are discrepancies in ageing animals using incremental analysis, especially in animals over eight years old. The actual process of counting layers (discussed at length in Chapter 4) is also open to a great deal of subjectivity, as is acknowledged by Miller (1974) who writes "histological examination of annuli in the dental cementum is a satisfactory technique for age determination of caribou. Ages assigned in this way are not exact due to problems of interpretation." Miller used a large modern population of animals and found difficulty with interpretation for ageing animals. Seasonality is more difficult to interpret than age assessment, so as more researchers become aware of the problems associated with cementum analysis, they would be rash to assume that accurate seasonal information can be obtained easily using this method.

More specifically, four main factors have been identified which contribute substantially towards the inaccuracy of this method. They are: the resorption of cementum; the existence of "false" (or "split" or "secondary") increments; the unevenness of cementum distribution over the tooth; and the problem of inconsistent terminology. In the remainder of this section, these four factors will be considered in turn. It should be noted in particular that the first three factors become especially problematic when only a fragment of the whole tooth is available: although it is clearly desirable that archaeological material should be preserved whenever possible, it seems extremely unlikely that any meaningful determination of age and seasonality can be made from such an isolated fragment.

An additional factor which needs to be considered when using incremental analysis in an archaeological context is taphonomy. It is often assumed that little will affect cementum once it has been mineralized, and that it will therefore remain unchanged in the ground. This optimistic point of view is challenged by work of Turner (1977). He examined the teeth of North American sheep, some of whose skulls had been picked up by field personnel from mountain ranges, and had thus been exposed to weathering conditions. He observed that incisors from weathered skulls showed a loss of annular definition. Klevezal (1996) had difficulty examining a mole skull that had been kept dry for 40 years. The effect of taphonomy should not be ignored and was shown to have a serious consequence on fauna from archaeological sites (Sørensen 1983). Further experiments should be undertaken to understand the effect on cementum of different conditions. Ideally teeth would be buried for a length of time in different environments, and then analyzed.

Cementum resorption

Though it has been claimed that cementum is rarely resorbed, or that where it is, the resorption tends to be localised (Stallibrass 1982, Lieberman and Meadow 1992), cementum, as noted above, is highly adaptive and the cells responsible for producing or removing cementum are provoked by changes in the health, function or distribution of any of the tissues in the periodontium (Jones, in Osborn 1981). As this is the case it is unrealistic to assume that resorption does not take place, or that a researcher should not be aware of it. Jones (in Osborn 1981) noted that both cementum and precement are resorbed and that resorption is most likely to follow a resting phase, to be found on the thicker apical region, and to be associated with an increase or change in the stress placed on a tooth. Resorption may also affect part of the dentine wall (Klevezal 1995) and therefore could affect the first band and thus invalidate any seasonality interpretation.
Keiss (1969) noted resorption in cementum of Elk. He observed that, because of resorption and repair on some teeth, layers could not be seen or counted readily in all areas of the cementum.

The causes of resorption are not properly understood: possible factors which may give rise to it include:

- An underlying disturbance in the function of the ductless gland. After the removal of the pressure resorptions are repaired by deposition of new cementum, fully restoring the contour of the root (Scott and Symons 1977).
- Occlusal trauma, when a single tooth or a group of teeth carry an abnormal amount of masticatory stress.
- Damage to the periodontal membrane (Bloom and Fawcett 1962 after Hemming 1969).

After the stress causing resorption is removed, the resorptions are generally repaired by the deposition of fresh cementum in all but the most severe cases. In human teeth, the repaired area is protected by an outer layer of cementoid tissue which is highly resistant to resorption (Sicher 1966 after Grimsdell 1973, Osborn 1981).

Root resorption is often manifested as reversal lines, which are scalloped in appearance and may be coated with a thin highly mineralized layer (Osborn 1981). This type of "layer" could easily be misinterpreted if the researcher were not familiar with the appearance of cementum layers, thus adding to the confusion of interpretation.

False/Split/Secondary increments

Rice (1980) carried out experiments to establish the influences of irregular cementum layers, and found that three types of irregular bands or lines could give rise to errors in counting the layers: false, split, and compound annuli. Rice studied 274 White-tailed deer and 250 Mule deer. In this sample he found that true increments are hard to distinguish from irregular increments, which occurred in half of the incisors aged over two and a half years.

False annuli appear as distinct individual layers on the anterior and posterior portions of the root, but become granular towards the root tip and disappear completely at the root apex. **Split annuli** appear as individual layers of equal width (see also Lockard 1972), but join into a single layer at or near the root apex. **Compound annuli** appear as a single layer on both sides of the root, but separate into two distinct layers near the root apex. By contrast, regular or **true annuli** are present as a single distinct layer on both the anterior and posterior root portions, and at the apex. Lockard (1972) and Grue and Jensen (1979) have suggested another type of line that can be identified within cementum layering, "resorption lines" that are the result of resorption and repair of the cementum in some areas.

Miller (1974) noted in his study of caribou that longitudinal sections are essential to expose the maximum number of annuli and therefore allow the observer to determine "more accurately the origins of annuli and the splitting, merging or phasing out of annulus along the course of the cementum. It is possible to miss such changes in the annulus when transverse sections are used"

Pike-Tay (1995), studying caribou, notes that in the cases where irregular layers were seen, they could not be linked to sex differences, but could be identified at the same area on different teeth from the same individual. This would seem to suggest that irregular layers are a consequence of an internal mechanism rather than of damage or mechanical stress, since such external factors would be unlikely to be evenly represented across the teeth. She also notes (Pike-Tay 1991) that by taking a complete longitudinal section and examining the entire length it is quite easy to recognize secondary lines as they are not continuous around the section. There are therefore obvious difficulties in examining only a small area of a tooth.

The causes of secondary increments are not clearly understood: this is connected to the general lack of understanding of the causes of cementum layering. Specifically, some authors have claimed that the secondary lines in deer may be double winter rest lines or rut lines (Low and Cowan 1963). Red deer stags accumulate fat during the summer and lose up to 20% of their body weight in the rut (Clutton-Brock, Guinness and Albon 1982). It is therefore assumed that, if nutrition is a cause of secondary lines, these would be marked in Red deer stags. Reimers and Norby (1968) also claimed to observe rut lines, but only in males from very good ranges. Ratcliffe and Mayle (1992) noted that in adult Roe deer bucks there are very often fine discontinuous lines, which they attribute to the rut, within the white bands. Aitken (1975) noted that in Roe deer, thick white bands are occasionally interrupted by a narrow, darker layer, which he suggested may be associated with lactation, which takes place from May to August-September: however, he goes on to note that a similar pattern was observed in four Roe bucks that he examined, which he attributes to the rut. A castrate three year old male doesn't demonstrate secondary lines of this type, which may suggest a hormonal reason for these additional lines. Douglas (1970) noted secondary lines in a population of New Zealand Red deer.

Miller (1974) noted that when double rest lines occurred in Caribou they were present in every year but the first, and in some cases only duplicated for a number of years. He concluded that no causal pattern could be established and that the low incidence of the condition did not justify further exploration. Likewise Omar (1992) studied a unique collection ofl13 known aged Red deer teeth from Rum with known life histories and sex, and concluded that there was no connection between secondary increments and the rut or lactation.

Mitchell (1967) in his study of Red deer noted an extra translucent band was associated with the time of the mating season (late September to mid October) in 180 (or about 25%) of the 800 mature stags examined. These bands were much narrower than winter/spring translucent lines, and divided each summer/autumn band into a broad and a narrow segment.

Even if rut lines could be established conclusively, it would only take us a little nearer to understanding causes of layering. One explanation would be hormonal, another would be that deer eat far less during the rut and therefore this could be a nutritional anomaly. Equally, given the reduced food intake, these rest lines could be the result of reduced stress on the teeth.

Kay (1974, after Lockard 1972) observed that split and false annuli on the sides of teeth generally converge and that they should be considered as a single annulus. He adds that false annuli occur in two forms. One form is near the outer edge of the cementum pad in the area between the roots and these undulate as finely denticulate lines, which are sometimes double. The second form is found at the interface between types of cementum, which integrate to form a band.

Whatever their cause, it is not disputed that secondary, or false, increments exist and provide a problem in interpretation: for what one researcher may identify as a secondary line, another may interpret as a primary.

The unevenness of cementum distribution

Several authors have pointed out the difficulties that arise from the unevenness of cementum distribution over the tooth. Thus, for example, Hemming (1969), studying Dall sheep, noted that "since the thickness of the cementum layer differs from place to place on the root of the tooth, saggital sections of the entire root proved to be the most satisfactory". Craighead, Craighead and McCutchen (1970), studying the Grizzly bear, "frequently prepared several slides before one was obtained that clearly showed all the growth layers". They "found it necessary to view sections along the entire length of the cementum". They observe that "cement deposition takes place over the entire root, but is thickest near the outer edge of the root tip. Localized thickenings of cement best show the sequence of layering." The implication of this final sentence is that one would default to this area when looking for the area of best fit, even though there is no reason to assume that it is any more accurate than other areas from which it differs.

Pike-Tay (1995) studied 348 Caribou from the Kaminuriak population, measuring the widths of increments at different sites of acellular cementum from the teeth of an individual. She concluded that there were differences in the widths which appeared to be neither predictable nor systematic. She adds that this may be a consequence of mechanical error in specimen preparation and data recording, rather than actual variation within the tooth. She claims that cementum is deposited at a regular rate only in areas of acellular cementum.

Omar (1992), studying 113 known aged Red deer from Rum, noted that not every incremental layer extends to the edge of the cementum and that the layers converge and become narrower at the edges of the specimen.

Aitken (1975) examined five known aged Roe deer from Dorset and observed that in a seven year old the seven bands were poorly defined owing to the scant development of the intervening zones of acellular cementum. Notably, the bands he identified were not continuous across the cut face of the cementum, so that in some places only six lines could be identified.

Pollitt (1993) studied cementum in human teeth and observed that layers are most distinct approximately half way down the length of the root. She noted that the distinction between the layers varied along the length of the root.

Shapiro (1995) examined and photographed a sample of 28 cattle tooth sections (11 of known age) under SEM. She noted that the clearest bands and lines were "limited to the cervical third of the root."

Willey (1974) studied bears and found that "although cement deposition is most dense near the top of the root, the area immediately adjacent to the crown of the tooth provided the easiest readings, particularly in bears younger than eight years. The same area however, is of almost no value for age determination of older bears." This could suggest that once the tooth has erupted, the area near the crown is no longer laying down cementum and that incremental analysis in this area is therefore not applicable for older animals. It is not clear at what age this would become an issue in most mammals.

Foley (1986) examined tropical ungulates and noted difficulties in ageing tropical mammals because the cementum deposition is frequently continuous and not marked by layering.

Additionally, with the difficulties of preservation of archaeological material, it would be difficult to establish if the area near the crown had less cementum than other areas because of lack of preservation of the increments or because of the age of the animal.

These doubts reinforce the need for a clear understanding of cementum. Given that incremental layers vary across the tooth, it seems clear that the "real" layering cannot be identified until the causes of "false" increments are understood. The most common approach seems to be to study the "area of best fit", although what it fits best with is not clear. This approach may allow approximate ageing, but not seasonality determination. Very often, the pad cementum (which is cellular) and the apical cementum are used for analysis, but these areas have their own interpretative problems, although some success was achieved by Mitchell (1963) using the pad cementum of red deer. Pike-Tay (1991) emphasizes that it is imperative that the entire root surface is scanned to ensure that one is reading the primary lines correctly.

The need for a known-aged sample

Given the plethora of difficulties and uncertainties described above, it is essential that any estimates of the age or season of death of animals from cementum incremental analysis should be based upon controlled studies of modern fauna of known age from analogous environments. This is, of course, particularly important before valuable archaeological specimens are sectioned. The need for having experience in the method of thin section preparation and an understanding of cementum has been stressed by many researchers (for example, Pike-Tay 1991, Burke 1992, Lieberman and Meadow 1992, Beasley, Brown and Legge 1992, Gordon 1991, Gasaway, Harkness and Rausch 1978, Miller 1974, Erickson and Seliger 1969, Thomas and Bandy 1973, Rice 1980), but has been observed by very few, as the following table illustrates:

Author	Species	Known aged	Modern Control	Seasons represented	Archaeological teeth sectioned
Beasley 1987	Red deer	None	None	NA	5
Beasley 1987	Horse	None	None	NA	2
Beasley et al 1992	Cattle	25	47	Unknown	"a very large sample"
Burke.A.1995	Horse	None	40	April, May	101
Lieberman 1990	Mountain gazelle	None	20	Feb,April,May, July,Aug,Oct,Nov, Dec	3
Landon 1993	Cow, pig, goat	None	6	June, Oct, Sept, Feb	77
Pike-Tay. A. 1991	Red deer	17	17	Oct,Nov,Dec,May	150
Kierdorf 1995	Reindeer	None	None	NA	4
Saxon and Higham 1968	Ovine	12	12	Two months only	6
Kay 1974	White tailed deer	None	None	NA	28
Coy, Jones & Turner 1982	Cattle	Approximate	25 jaws	Three months	64
Burke & Castanet 1995	Horse	No	16	Nine months	104
Gordon 1988	Caribou	62	62	April,June, July, Nov, Dec	447
Spiess 1989	Zebra, Hartebeest	None	None	NA	67

Table 2: Modern control samples in archaeological cementum incremental studies.

The meaning of the term *known-aged* also has a variety of interpretations. Some researchers use it to describe teeth that they believe they have aged correctly, and while this may be justified for very young animals for which the eruption sequence provides an accurate assessment of age, the term should nevertheless be qualified. For example, Gordon (1988) states that he uses 62 modern known aged teeth, and then tests his technique on 'known-aged' teeth from Barrenland and French archaeological sites. In my opinion, the term should only be used when animals are tagged at birth.

Jensen and Nielsen (1968) studied 500 foxes using decalcified sections, and concluded that accurate ages can only be obtained after a great deal of experience with known aged material. Similarly, Smuts, Anderson and Austin (1978) examined 43 African Lions of known age, and, while finding a good correlation between age and increment counts, comment that "had the known-age material not been available for the present study, interpretation of the pattern of cement apposition could not have been achieved".

Some researchers use tooth wear and eruption, supposedly providing accurate ages, to calibrate incremental analysis (Koike & Ohtaishi 1985). Tooth wear itself requires subjective judgments, and certainly does provide an accurate ageing of every animal: it is certainly not a sufficiently precise method to use as a basis for calibrating incremental analysis. For more detail on ageing by tooth wear, see Chapters 5 and 6.

Even if a large modern known-aged sample can be obtained, there can still be difficulties, particularly in the archaeological context, in correlating it with the population of unknown age as regards environment, behaviour, diet, and other such features.

Discussion

Cementum is a complex material that needs to be understood before any analysis is attempted. The causes of cementum layering are not known, and there are many unproven theories that have been put forward. Secondary lines and bands are often seen, but the causes of these are also not understood. Some researchers even acknowledge their existence but choose to ignore them (Gordon 1988).

Once the tooth is deposited in the ground, the potential for destruction of the cementum, particularly individual bands or lines that are only a few microns thick, is high. Koike and Ohtaishi (1985) examined archaeological teeth from in situ jaws and isolated teeth using observation methods and cementum increments. They noted that incremental layers of excavated teeth were more difficult to read than modern material. They add that the images of layers were unclear due to the prior preservation especially near the surface of the cementum. Lieberman (1992) also demonstrates some concern over the preservation of the structure of archaeological teeth, particularly the loss of the outer edge of the cementum, which is required for seasonality determination. Frison, Wilson and Wilson (1976) attempted analysis on 6500 year old bison; they were unsuccessful because chemical alteration had disrupted the structure, reducing the visibility of the increments. Kay (1974) found that of 28 sections originally produced, only 20 were suitable for analysis. Burke (1995) found that of her archaeological sample, 75% demonstrated increments that could be observed. It is worth noting that if the sample is reduced by 25% because no increments can be observed, that it is unlikely that the remainder of the sample are all perfect. Very little research has been attempted on known aged material, specifically known aged material which covers all seasons, and whose provenance is close to the environment of the archaeological material.

The evidence is that it would be meaningless to attempt incremental analysis on single isolated teeth from archaeological sites, particularly fragments of teeth, regardless of the sectioning/examination method being employed and despite the suggestions of some authors (Burke 1993, Beasley 1987).

Chapter Two
Age and Seasonality Determination - a review

This chapter provides a review of some of the most important work, both by archaeologists and by wildlife biologists, on the use of cementum incremental analysis to determine the age and season of death of an animal. Before embarking upon this review, I shall explain the importance of age and seasonality determination to archaeologists, and survey some of the other techniques which have been used for seasonality determination.

1. AGE DETERMINATION

Age determination of animals from archaeological sites is of great interest to archaeologists. Age determination of single animals, although of some interest, is less important than building age profiles for as many of the faunal remains as possible. In this way, the archaeologist can move towards understanding and interpreting the economies of the site, whether it is a hunting or a domestic site. By ageing animals killed on known hunting sites it is possible to identify whether the kills are selective, seasonal, or natural (for example through some catastrophic event). A random distribution of the ages of death suggests that hunters were picking off those animals which were easier to kill, or that certain animals were more abundant at a given time. As regards domestic sites, age profiles can help us to understand how the fauna was managed or herded. Economy plays a large part in the age and sex of the animal. Kills of young males may suggest meat eating, while older female animals may suggest secondary products such as milk or skin. It may even be possible, in conjunction with seasonality analysis, to identify the transition from hunting to farming if one can identify an early herding of what were once hunted species (Davis 1983).

Wildlife biologists use a variety of different techniques to identify age profiles of live species. There are two main classes of age determination, relative and absolute. Relative methods are often based on tooth wear, eye lens weight, and other measurements, whereas absolute ages are obtained through biological tissue study. Many of these techniques are not applicable to archaeological fauna, since they are based on soft tissue study: for example, body weight, eye lens dry weight, or overall body condition. Some other methods, such as epiphyseal fusion (discussed in more detail below) can occasionally be applied to archaeological fauna, if the deposition of the bone has allowed for its preservation. However, this technique is in any case limited in use, since it can only be applied to young animals, and the timing of fusion is affected by health and nutritional stress, factors which would be impossible to identify in archaeological material. Epiphyseal fusion has been used to successfully age animals from archaeological sites (Bull and Payne 1982, Bullock and Rackham 1982). Horn cores have also been examined for ageing animals from archaeological sites (Armitage 1982).

Tooth eruption and wear is commonly used for ageing by wildlife biologists and archaeologists alike (for details see Chapter 5). These methods have also been used with some success to determine seasonality (Legge and Rowley-Conwy 1988).

2. SEASONALITY DETERMINATION

The importance of seasonality

Seasonality is about the way in which human behaviour and activity is influenced by the natural variation of the seasons. Anthropologists are aware of the roles that seasonal variation plays in human physiology, geography, demography and economy (Cross 1989). Dispersion and aggregation of populations is commonly a result of seasonal fluctuations in food resource availability (Monks 1981). In developing models of hunter/gatherer settlement and subsistence in prehistory, we must proceed from the valid premise that prehistoric hunter-gatherers changed their settlement size, location, group composition and thus their social morphology in keeping with the annual cycle of seasons. Information regarding prehistoric seasonality then provides insight into critical areas of human social and economic life at a regional scale (Pike-Tay 1991). In order to assess the economic sub-system of any given culture, it is essential to define the variety of site-types, their function, extent, and the duration and season of occupation. Such a procedure is a prerequisite to any attempt to define the parameters of the linked social sub-system (Coutts and Higham 1971).

Archaeologists tend to approach the study of seasonality in two ways. First, by having a knowledge of the natural environment they can model seasonal variation in available resources. Second, they can accumulate data from individual sites that is related to seasonal use of the site and create an aggregate picture. Both of these approaches express seasonal resource availability or use as a single annual cycle (Cross 1989).

Saxon and Higham (1968) showed how resource procurement is highly seasonal amongst most groups. Dispersion and aggregation of populations is commonly a result of seasonal fluctuations in food resource availability. A site may be occupied all year round, sporadically throughout the year, or for one specific season. In hunting and gathering communities seasonal availability of resources could dictate whether a site is a hunting site, a home base, a source of raw material, or a trading post.

Seasonal indicators are used to test predications generated by models of settlement and subsistence: for example the degree of mobility of the settlement system predicted by herd following can be tested against patterns of site occupation (Burke 1992). It is important to understand prehistoric peoples' seasonal movement as this restricted permanent settlement, family size and material culture (Gordon 1988).

Seasonality is therefore of great interest to archaeologists - so great in fact that debates have raged for years over the seasonality of some sites, such as Star Carr in Yorkshire. Some forty years after the original excavation of this site by Clark between 1949 and 1951, there are still doubts about its seasonal occupation (Clark 1954, 1972, Caulfield 1978, Jacobi 1978, Wheeler 1978, Pitts 1979, Andersen, Byrd, Elson, Mcguire, Mendoza, Staski and White 1981, Grigson 1981, Price 1982, Legge and Rowley-Conwy 1988, Carter 1997, 1998). Seasonality is essential for deeper understanding of the character of human occupation and economic activities at the site. Establishing the seasonality of this site is of great importance, since the majority of interpretations of seasonal economic patterns in the 8th Millennium BC have been built around it. Because of the abundance of data available from Star Carr, the site is central to debates surrounding the nature of early Mesolithic settlement in Europe.

Methods for determining seasonality

Various methods have been used to determine the seasonality of archaeological sites, so many, indeed, that Monks (1981) suggests that seasonality should be a subject area in its own right. None of these techniques is definitive: they can only be seen as providing evidence for occupation of the site at a given season. Some techniques, such as incremental analysis of cementum, claim to be accurate, but such techniques are also beset with problems that hinder a complete understanding of seasonality. These include incremental growth of mollusc shell (Clark 1980, Hancock 1984, Koike 1979), and the examination of fish scales and otoliths (Casteel 1976, Pannella 1980).

In the remainder of this section, brief descriptions will be given of the principal methods of faunal analysis for seasonality determination.[1]

Though faunal remains are often used to indicate season of occupation of a site, there is always the issue that a lack of remains for other seasons does not necessarily mean that the site was not occupied at other times of the year. Absence of proof is not proof of absence (Davis 1987). Also, even if the time of death of the animal can be established, it does not necessarily mean that the animal was killed at that site at that time.

[1] Other methods such as the presence or absence of floral species are also used to determine site seasonality but have not been examined in this study.

1. Antler morphology

In most cervids, only males carry antlers: the exception is reindeer where both the males and females carry them. Antlers are very dense and highly mineralized, and are therefore preserved nearly as well as bone (Monks 1981). Antlers follow a cycle of growth, maturity, and shedding at given times of the year depending on the species. The presence of shed or unshed antlers have therefore been used to identify the season of occupation of sites. In some cases antler may indicate seasonal use, for example the unworked Roe deer antler at Star Carr Yorkshire (Legge and Rowley-Conwy 1988). The principal difficulty with this technique is that antler was a valuable raw material which would remain on the landscape for quite a long period of time. It is therefore likely that antlers would travel with hunter gatherers, and may not have been deposited at the season of use. This was almost certainly the case for the worked antler frontlets from Star Carr in Yorkshire which had been lightened and perforated for attachment to the head of a hunter-gatherer (Legge and Rowley-Conwy 1988). This may be an extreme example but, as has already been explained, antler was a source of raw material and therefore ascribing strict seasonal use to their presence or absence should be done with care.

2. Osteoporosis

Osteoporosis is the pitting of long bones in birds, which may indicate egg-laying, moulting, or nutritional stress. It has also been observed in white tailed deer at times of antler regeneration, pregnancy, and nutritional stress (Monks 1981). However, pinpointing the exact timing of such events can be difficult, and there is no clear way of distinguishing between different events which may give rise to osteoporosis.

3. Tooth wear and eruption

If one knows the season when animals are born and the sequence that is followed in tooth wear and eruption, it may be possible to identify the season of death of very young animals. Because of its restricted applicability to young animals, this technique has limited use in building seasonal profiles. For a detailed account see Chapters 5, 6, and 7.

4. Epiphyseal fusion

Epiphyseal fusion is a commonly used method of seasonal estimation. Many bones found on archaeological sites are ends or fragments of shafts. The cartilage which joins the articular surface to the main body of a bone slowly ossifies (Monks 1981). The ends can be classified according to the state of fusion of its epiphysis, as unfused (juvenile) or fused (adult) (Davis 1983). Monks (1981) claims that there are difficulties in using this approach as authors do not distinguish between (a) epiphyseal fusion schedules on the same element from different species, (b) fusion schedules on different elements of the same species and (c) different ages at which fusion occurs on bones having more than one epiphyses. He goes on to point out that fusion happens over a long period of time and is affected by nutritional stress. An additional problem, which he does not mention, is that as the bone is not completely ossified there may be problems of preservation in the ground.

Davis (1987) provides a table of the approximate ages of epiphysial fusion for a number of species, pointing out that these ages do vary between species.

5. Fish
Fish grow throughout their lives with very little remodelling of their hard tissue (Davis 1987). Parts of their skeletons exhibit alternating wide and narrow rings associated with seasonal fluctuations in growth, related to breeding, and to variations in water temperature, day length and food availability. This layering is seen in otoliths, scales, vertebral centra, and operculars. Seasonal changes are found in species living where there are seasonal changes in water temperature.

6. Oxygen isotope analysis
This method was well described by Shackleton (1973). It exploits the temperature related uptake of the oxygen isotope in marine shells (Monks 1981). This method uses oxygen isotope variation to measure the temperature of the water when the growing edge of the shell was being produced (Davis 1987).

7. Presence or absence of seasonally available species
This method is based upon the presence or absence of migratory birds, mammals, and fish. The underlying assumption is that their remains were brought onto the site by humans, and that they did not die naturally. This includes the assumption that the remains were deposited at the time of use, and hadn't been preserved for a period of time or brought in from another site some distance away. Given that animals are a source of a variety of raw materials, such as bone, fur and sinew, it is not unreasonable to argue that remains found were not necessarily deposited in a given four month period to indicate a season of use, as explained above in the case of antler.

8. Incremental structures
This method is based upon growth rates. Incremental structures can be affected by temperature, changes in nutrition, hormonal changes, migration (giving rise to seasonal changes in temperature), food availability, and breeding cycles. Varying rates of growth can be identified, with the most recent growth increments resting on the previous growth layer.

Mammal teeth and bones often exhibit incremental structures (Klevezal and Kleinberg 1969, Laws 1952, 1962, Klevezal 1996).

3. HISTORY OF INCREMENTAL ANALYSIS

Tooth increments occur in nearly all mammals: temperate, tropical, and polar; land and sea; those that hibernate, and those that remain active all year. They are also found in amphibian and reptilian teeth and bones (Gordon 1991). The analysis of these increments is commonly regarded as one of the most accurate techniques for determining seasonality. The majority of research has been focused on teeth rather than bone, because of inherent difficulties in the analysis of bone, which is remodelled throughout life as it adapts to functional influences, and is subject to resorption (Stallibrass 1982). Teeth are very robust, and are thus more likely to remain in the ground; there is an assumption that they are resistant to abrasion, fire, and dissolution (Gordon 1991) but as Maltby (1982) suggests, the number of isolated teeth on archaeological sites would indicate that they were once part of jaws that had not survived in the ground. Although this is true for the main bulk of teeth, it is not necessarily the case for cementum (see Chapter 1 for further discussion of this point). Because of their robustness, teeth are abundant on many archaeological sites, where other elements which might be used as seasonal indicators may not remain. Furthermore, many archaeologists have been attracted to incremental analysis of teeth because they believe that the analysis can be performed on isolated teeth, or even on tooth fragments (Pike-Tay 1991, Beasley 1987). It is my belief that the problems associated with incremental analysis are compounded when dealing with isolated teeth to such an extent that any such results obtained should be treated with the greatest caution (a more extended discussion can be found in Chapter 1).

Examination and analysis has been performed on both dentine and cementum of teeth. Despite the popularity of ageing animals using dentine incremental analysis (Klevezal and Kleinberg 1966, Morris 1972, Casteel 1976, Klevezal 1996), it is limited in usefulness because, once the pulp cavity has been filled, no more dentine can be laid down. Most mammal teeth cease growing in length in the first to third year of life. The pulp of the tooth gets narrower, remaining wide in the middle of the tooth. During the next years the tooth wall gets thicker owing to deposition of new dentine layers until the pulp cavity is filled up (Klevezal 1996). Thus the technique is not applicable to older animals. It has also been noted that dentine often has confusing accessory lines (Morris 1972). These would be similar to the secondary, spilt or false increments identified in cementum.

There is a very long history of research into incremental structures, especially by wildlife biologists, who need to understand life histories for management purposes. They have for many years been studying both dentine and cementum increments for age and season of death (Gordon (1991) has references dating back to Retzius, von A. in 1837). Both full and selective bibliographies have been compiled by Klevezal (1996), Casteel (1973), Gordon (1984, 1991), Monks (1981), and Stallibrass (1982). Of these authors, it appears that only Klevezal and Gordon have actually attempted incremental analysis themselves. Methodological work of the highest quality has been documented by Klevezal and Kleinberg (1969), Grue and Jensen (1979), Lieberman et al. (1990), and Klevezal (1996). Further details on methodological issues are given in Chapter 3.

Many cementum incremental studies were performed during the 1960s and 1970s. Although the following is not an exhaustive bibliography (see Klevezal 1996 and Gordon 1991 for these), it gives an indication of the scale of interest, and of the diversity of mammals being studied. One common theme amongst these papers is that no standard terminology, method, or approach has been adopted. (Armstrong 1965a, 1965b, Bovidae; Gilbert 1966, White tailed deer; Ransome 1966, White tailed deer; Greer and Yeager 1967, Elk (wapiti); Lowe 1967, Red deer from Rum; Mitchell 1967, Red deer; Olson, 1967, White tailed deer; Spinage 1967, Waterbuck; Prior 1968, Roe deer; Reimers and Nordby 1968, Reindeer; Saxon and Higham 1968, sheep; Erickson and Seliger 1969, Mule deer; Kiess 1969, Elk; Klevezal and Kleinberg 1969, mammals; McCutchen 1969, Pronghorns; Wolfe 1969, Moose; Douglas 1970, Red deer; Erickson et al. 1970, Mule deer; Gilbert and Stolt 1970, White-tailed deer; Robinette and Archer 1971, Thomson's gazelle; Brokx 1972, White-tailed deer; Lockard 1972, White-tailed deer; Grimsdell 1973, African buffalo; Thomas and Bandy 1973, Black-tailed deer; Kay 1974, White-tailed deer; Miller 1974, Caribou; Stoddart 1974, Roe deer; Aitken 1975, Roe deer; Steenkamp 1975, wildlife in general; Rudge 1976, sheep; Spinage 1976a, tropical mammals; Spinage 1976b, Grant's gazelle; Turner 1977, North American sheep; Gasaway et al. 1978, Moose; Grue and Jensen 1979, terrestrial mammals).

In the last fifteen years or so there has been far more use of cementum incremental analysis, and a greater willingness to accept some of the limitations associated with it. Equally, more use has been made of the technique for application to archaeological material. Focusing on the major works, I will outline briefly some of the uses of the technique and results that have been obtained.

Ungulate specific research

There are many papers relating to ungulates (Eidermann 1932, Raesfield 1957, Sergeant and Pimlott 1959, Low and Cowan 1963, McEwan 1963, Mitchell 1963, 1967, Gilbert 1964, 1966, Ransom 1966, Greer and Yeager 1967, Lowe 1967, Spinage 1967, Prior 1968, Reimers and Nordby 1968, Saxon and Higham 1968, Sohn 1968, Erickson and Seliger 1969, Keiss 1969, McCutchen 1969, Wolfe 1969, Douglas 1970, Flook 1970, Gilbert and Stolt 1970, Brokx 1972, Lockard 1972, Thomas and Bandy 1973, Kay 1974, Miller 1974a, 1974b, Stoddart 1974, Aitken 1975, Steenkamp 1975, Rudge 1976, Spinage 1976a, 1976b, Turner 1977, Gasaway, Harkness and Rausch 1978, Rice 1980, Coy, Jones and Turner 1982, Koike and Ohtaishi 1985, Spiess 1985, Beasley 1987, Gordon 1988, Lieberman, Deacon and Meadow 1990, Lieberman and Meadow 1991). Many of the results of these papers and the issues raised in them are discussed in other chapters of this study. Below is an outline of a few of these papers to provide an overview of previous research.

Eidmann had little success with the study of Red deer dentine for age determination in 1932 and 1933. However, later research helped to move the study forward. Sergent and Pilmott (1959) sectioned moose incisor teeth and discovered that cementum increments may occur before eruption. They also noted that the differences and contrasts between bands and lines are dependent on the uses of reflected and transmitted light.

Low and Cowan (1963) studied Mule deer and observed that possible rut lines could be identified. These would now be classed as secondary, split or false increments (see Chapter 1).

McEwan (1963) looked at Barren Ground Caribou and found that it was necessary to add a year to the opaque increment count to obtain accurate ages, though he observed that increments also occurred in both an eight month old calf and a three month old calf. If the increments were clear in a three month old calf this would suggest that there was no need to add a year onto the final count to obtain accurate ages. They claimed that this difference may have been due to difference in nutrition and daylight hours. It is interesting to note that even at this time there were already differences in opinion as to how the increments were being formed, with little attempt at standardization.

Mitchell (1963) examined Red deer teeth from Scotland for ageing purposes. He looked at wear and molar pad cementum thickness using reflected light. He found that there was some correlation between age at death and cementum layers formed on the pad. In 1967, Mitchell examined teeth of over 3000 Red deer from Scotland, collected over six years. This sample included animals from natural deaths such as starvation and avalanches. Of this sample, 22 were of known age with 9 being between one and two years old, 8 being between two and three years old, 3 being between three and four years old and the remaining two seventeen and a half and nineteen and a half years old. He concluded that cementum growth is related to the rate of wear and is much greater on the cheek teeth than on incisors and canines.

Mitchell allowed many samples to rot naturally before examination in order to make it easier to extract them from the jaws. Lower first molars were used and the fine structure of the dental cementum was examined using sections between 50 and 100 microns thick, and viewed under a transmitted light microscope. The sections were made using a hacksaw and ground using carborundum paper. For routine examination of the pad cementum facial sections were used and viewed under reflected light with a dissecting microscope. Mitchell found a correlation between the number of layers and the age of the animal in all but one of these specimens.

Interestingly it is the oldest animal that shows the weakest correlation. It is unfortunate that most of the other animals were very young and therefore could have been aged equally accurately using eruption and tooth wear.

Lowe (1967) also studied Red deer from Rum using various techniques including tooth wear, dentine analysis and cementum incremental analysis. He looked at the root pad cementum and concluded that increments are irregular and poor for age estimation.

Moore et al (1995) studied 50 known aged Fallow deer jaws from Phoenix Park, Dublin, aged between 4 and 131 months. They compared five different techniques for ageing: tooth eruption, incisor height, molar height, molar wear and layers in dental cementum. They measured the incisor height of 36 of the animals from the lowest point of the gum line to the highest point of the crown. Molar heights were taken from the enamel-cementum junction to the highest point on the mesial-buccal cusp on 41 of the animals, and molar wear scores were determined for 48 animals. 30 molars were then sectioned. Molar wear score was assessed using the Brown and Chapman method (1990). The cementum layers were counted on the dental pad of the first molar. The sections were examined three times on different occasions. If the readings were not identical a fourth reading was taken. If three of the four agreed, then that was the figure that was used. If no three readings agreed, a fifth reading was made and a median figure used. They found that incisor height was the most accurate method (90%), while cementum incremental analysis was only 53% accurate, and molar wear scores were only 43% accurate. Overall they claim that the age of the animal does not affect the accuracy of any of these methods. They also concluded, "It is assumed that in higher latitudes the so–called winter band of cementum is associated with a growth check". However, populations differ in the extent to which individuals develop cementum layers. Within species, populations in areas with more continental climates generally have a clearer, more definite banding pattern than those from oceanic climates (Leader and Williams 1979).

Thus there may be large numbers of animals in which distinct layers cannot be detected. This adds to the overall instability of cementum as an accurate indicator of age and season, given the many factors which can affect the accuracy of the technique and the tissue itself.

Although Moore et al found that incisor height was the most accurate method of ageing, incisors very rarely survive in the jaw on archaeological sites, and cannot therefore be used as an accurate method for ageing archaeological fauna. The Brown and Chapman scheme was developed using young known aged animals and was therefore not intended for use on a much older population. The scheme would not have been applicable to animals over six years, even if the environment that the animals were living in was the same: the low accuracy of the scoring scheme was therefore to be expected when applied to older specimens (see Chapter 6). Incisors of Mule deer were sectioned by Erickson and Seliger (1969), they concluded that "only persons experienced through the study of known aged material or instruction by an experienced co-worker should use the technique". Rice (1980) who examined white tailed deer and mule deer incisors using incremental analysis reached a similar conclusion. He observed that true increments were hard to distinguish from irregular increments which occurred in half of the incisors over two and a half years old.

The low level of accuracy of cementum incremental analysis found by Moore et al (1995) and the difficulties experienced by Erickson and Seliger (1969) are in line with the results from this study (see Chapter 4).

Advantages and limitations of cementum incremental analysis

Given that there is such a long history of cementum incremental analysis, it is surprising that it was not until 1969 that the technique was first employed by archaeologists (namely Saxon and Higham 1969). It is also surprising, given the supposed accuracy of the method, that it has not been more widely applied to meaningful archaeological samples. A number of issues which affect the accuracy and reliability of cementum incremental analysis are presented in this study (see Chapters 1, 3, and 4).

The following table provides a summary of some of the advantages and limitations of cementum incremental analysis.

Proposed advantages of cementum analysis	Observed limitations of cementum analysis
Cementum is deposited throughout life of the animal (see Chapter 1)	
It can be applied to any mammal of any age or sex	Only accurately if a modern, known age population is available for testing.
Unlike bone, cementum is not easily resorbed.	Areas of resorption do occur, and experience is needed to identify these areas.
If used properly it can provide accurate age assessments	Analysis is subjective, and dependant on technique: examiner reliability is very poor.
It has a proven accuracy for some species (Klevezal 1996)	Little success has been achieved with other species (e.g. Lowe 1967).
Teeth survive well on archaeological sites.	The technique is destructive, and teeth need to be cut out of the jaw.
It is claimed that it can be applied to isolated teeth (Beasley 1986)	The outer edge of the cementum will probably not survive on isolated teeth.
	The timing of the formation of the first band or line is not always known.
	The neonatal line, first band/line and second band/ line are not always distinct and can lead to underestimates in age.
	The causes of incremental layers are not understood.

	Secondary lines/bands can cause inaccurate age assessments if not properly identified.
	The cementum is not evenly distributed around the root, and may be difficult to read in some areas.
	The older an animal is, the harder it is to distinguish clear incremental layers.
	Sectioning techniques differ and require expertise, and are very costly and time-consuming.

Table 3: Advantages and disadvantages of cementum incremental analysis.

Lieberman (1990) claims that there are four major problems that affect an investigator's ability to identify and interpret incremental structures in cementum:

1. **Unknown mechanisms**: lack of understanding of the causes of layering. It is therefore imperative not to assume that the technique works for all specimens or species.

2. **Sampling**: there are a number of unavoidable difficulties in analyzing cementum increments of teeth from archaeological contexts. Specimens must be well preserved and carefully handled to ensure retention of cementum layers. Even when the presence of the outer increment can be safely assumed, as in the case of firmly embedded teeth in the mandible or maxilla (or can be demonstrated by the presence of traces of the periodontal ligament in modern specimens), inner increments can be missing or severely collapsed, especially in old individuals or in small teeth (Klevezal and Kleinberg 1967, Kay 1989 after Lieberman 1990). Thus, in sections taken from teeth embedded in jaws (or with remnants of the periodontal ligament still attached), estimation of season of death for older individuals is more likely to be correct than is estimation of age at death. For interpretative purposes, care must be taken to use as many teeth as possible from any site or locus, and increment data should always be tested against other available information on age and seasonality.

3. **Specimen quality**: the resolution of cementum increments, particularly in the case of archaeological material, is sometimes poor. Teeth can be stained, fossilized, decalcified, or without most of their organic component, making it difficult to identify clearly all of the increments. Outer increments can be removed through abrasion, leading to false estimates of age and season of death. Lieberman et al suggest that only teeth embedded in bone be analyzed, and that they be carefully cut out with a small rotary saw if they must be removed from the bone.

4. **Investigator subjectivity**: the determination of age and season of death in most analyses is subjective, dependent upon the judgment of the individual investigator, and often affected by poor resolution of increments and uneven sample preparation. What one researcher might interpret under transmitted polarized light as an opaque increment may appear to another to be a false or split translucent band. It is thus necessary to develop protocols and techniques for recording, quantifying and presenting increment data that are as objective as possible.

Gordon (1989) has begun this effort with suggestions for standardized terminology which Lieberman uses in this paper.

Thus it is recognized that there are many limitations to cementum incremental analysis. In summary, cementum is a complex material and though it does demonstrate layering which has been broadly applied to ageing, it should be acknowledged that there is no understanding as to the cause of these increments and therefore more thought and care is necessary before any seasonality theory is applied.

Additionally different techniques will provide different problems, thus Klevezal (1996) can obtain accuracy in the ageing of some species (e.g. Red deer) using decalcified sections, that other researchers cannot using standard ground thin sectioning techniques (Lowe 1967). Decalcification is not applicable to archaeological material, as is explained in Chapter 3.

The sectioning technique is expensive and training is needed in the production of the thin section and in the analysis of the section when completed.

Modern control populations should always be used, although these can often be difficult to obtain (Pike-Tay 1991).

All of these considerations should be taken into account when reviewing the literature and attempting to understand why so many studies seemingly contradict each other.

Chapter Three
Sectioning Technique

1. BACKGROUND

A precise, repeatable thin section production method is imperative for accurate interpretation of the material being examined. "A major requirement in the interpretation of sections is an appreciation of the processes involved in their production (Clevedon Brown & Hilton 1979). It is therefore essential that any researcher wishing to examine thin sections for incremental analysis has either produced the section themselves or has a very good understanding of the process before analysis is undertaken. This is particularly important for archaeological material, which is too precious to take unnecessary risk with.

There are many different ways of preparing a tooth prior to performing incremental analysis. On the most basic level, wildlife biologists, particularly when working in the field, have been known to cut a tooth in half with a hacksaw, polish it on a pumice stone or emery paper, and then examine either the pad cementum or the cementum at the base of the roots to estimate age (Mitchell 1963, Aitken R.J. 1975, Ratcliffe and Mayle 1992, Rose H. pers. comm.). A rather more refined technique, often used for approximate age determination, is to prepare a thick section of the tooth for analysis under reflected light (Mitchell 1967, Douglas 1969, Omar 1992, Moore, Cahill, Kelly, & Hayden 1995).

Other techniques include the paraffin technique (Low and Cowan 1963, Adams & Watkins 1967, Thomas and Bandy 1973, Steenkamp 1975), the use of a cryostat to cut teeth after freezing (Crowe 1972) and celloidin techniques (Tumlison R., McDaniel 1983).

A commonly used method, both by wildlife and marine biologists, is the preparation of a thin section produced by decalcification (or demineralisation). The calcium phosphate minerals of enamel, dentine and cementum may be dissolved away using dilute acids (Hillson 1986). Decalcification can be achieved by one of four main methods: by the use of mineral acids; and or organic acids; or of organic buffers; or by the use of chelating agents (Clevedon Brown & Hilton 1979). Once decalcified the specimen is then embedded in wax, or frozen, sectioned on a microtome and stained before being viewed under transmitted light (McEwan E.H. 1963, Stoneberg R.P. 1966, Marks & Erickson 1966, Adams, L. & Watkins, S.G. 1967, Klevezal & Kleinenberg 1967, Reimers E. & Nordby O. 1968, Jensen & Nielsen 1968, Keiss R.E. 1969, Erickson J.A. & Seliger W.G. 1969, Craighead J.J., Craighead F.C. & McCutchen H.E. 1970, Lockard G.R. 1972, Grue H. & Jensen B. 1973, Willey C.H. 1974, Miller F. 1974, Allen S. H. 1974, Grue H. & Jensen B. 1976, Spinage, C.A. 1976, Kolb H, 1978, Turner 1977, Fogl and Mosby 1978, Roberts, J.D. 1978, Smuts, G.L., Anderson, J.L, & Austin, J.C. 1978, Hackett, E.J., Guynn D.C., & Jacobson, H.A 1979, Grue H. & Jensen B. 1979, Rice, L.A. 1980, Hillson 1986: Klevezal, G.A. & Pucek, Z. 1987). The stains are useful for demonstrating the presence of different tissue components (Hillson 1986). Hillson (1986) suggests that intact sections of teeth can be demineralised and stained in situ on the slide if required, and this may be of use for archaeological material. Clevedon Brown & Hilton (1979) provide an excellent summary of sectioning techniques.

Generally decalcification is not a suitable preparation technique for archaeological material due to the low collagen content. "Demineralisation has considerable disadvantages for archaeological material. Enamel is almost entirely mineral and is so effectively destroyed by the method. Demineralisation also eliminates all mineral structures in dentine and cementum. In this way information is lost from the specimens that cannot be replaced." (Hillson 1986). Spiess (1976) decalcified fragments of Zebra and Hartebeest teeth from the site of Lukenya Hill, dated to 18,000 years old, which led to complete dissolution of the samples. Coy J.P, Jones R.T. & Turner K.A. (1982), looking at cattle from Saxon sites, decalcified both the modern control sample and the archaeological sample of 87 mandible fragments of archaeological origin, only 37 of which provided acceptable sections. Demineralisation has been used by archaeologists to section their modern material, while the archaeological material was sectioned using standard ground techniques similar to the one described below (Saxon & Higham 1968, Beasley, Brown & Legge 1992). There are obvious difficulties when using two very different thin section methodologies to compare the same elements, especially as "the technique of preparation of thin sections can have significant effects on the interpretation of samples" (Lieberman & Meadow 1992). Klevezal (1996) states "it is difficult to compare data obtained from ground sections and from stained sections". McEwan (1962) examined the cementum of first incisor teeth from barren ground Caribou using reflected, transmitted and polarised light. He concluded that cementum increments were not detectable. However on one hundred incisor teeth that were sectioned using decalcification both dentine and cementum increments could be identified and counted. Given the many complications that are in any case inherent in section interpretation (discussed in detail in chapter 3), it seems unwise to add unnecessary complications. Using different sectioning methods on the modern control sample and the archaeological sample essentially allows for no direct comparison between the two populations.[1]

Although many archaeologists have applied, and continue to apply, thin sectioning techniques, very few of them

[1] The opposite of demineralisation is also possible. Organic material may be removed using strong alkalis to expose the mineral component by itself (Wells 1974).

have any length of experience or describe in any detail the methods used for the preparation and sectioning of samples, providing only a brief overview of technique applied: nor is any description commonly given of the location of the tooth at which the cementum is being studied, or the microscopical techniques employed to study it; nor is the terminology for describing what is seen through the microscope standard. As a result, the analysis described in such papers is not repeatable. Even those archaeologists who do provide more detailed information betray, on the whole, little understanding of the factors that might affect or damage the section, or change the likely view down the microscope. A poorly made section can reflect light, or give an illusion of depth, thereby distorting the increments viewed. This fact was also noted by Burke (1992), who wrote "the cut must be perpendicular to the cementum surface since the thickness of the increments will vary if viewed at an angle and because annuli may appear double due to an optical affect if viewed on a slant" (Pascal & Quere 1983, after Burke 1992). Omar (1992) studied 113 known aged red deer from Rum and found that solid sections give optical distortions that misrepresent the nature of the cementum bands.

Pike-Tay (1995) looked at 348 Caribou from the Kaminuriak population and after measuring the widths of increments at the sites of acellular cementum from different teeth of an individual concluded that there were differences in the widths and that these differences did not seem to be predictable or systematic. She adds that it is as likely to be the result of mechanical error during specimen preparation and data recording as it is of actual variation between teeth. This emphasises the need for accurate sectioning and experience in addition to an essential review of the causes of cementum layering.

Since the observation of increments is in itself open to a great deal of interpretative error (see Chapter 4), it is essential that the thin sections produced be of high quality, and that the method used to produce them be repeatable, so as to minimise the error which arises from technique, in turn minimising errors that are likely to arise in the interpretation of the section.

Given the many possible sources of errors outlined in this thesis, I would like to reiterate the need for researchers to be both more precise in their technique and more diligent in recording the details of it. Sectioning of archaeological material should not be attempted until the examiner has a complete understanding of sectioning techniques, microscopical techniques and an acceptable number of modern controls, for each species to be studied, has been examined.

This chapter records the details of the sectioning technique that I developed by a long process of trials, although it is very similar to previous work (Kay 1974, Gordon 1988, Pike-Tay 1991, Burke 1992, Lieberman & Meadow 1992). I undertook to examine in detail every aspect of thin section production, without taking anything for granted. Sectioning is a practical undertaking, and though basic understanding can be established through the literature, it is only by trial and error and a great deal of experience that a real understanding can be achieved.

The technique provides a repeatable method of producing high quality thin sections that can be produced to a preferred thickness (e.g. 30 microns), with part of the tooth being preserved for study as a thick section. I am very grateful to B. Harris in the department of Geology of the University of Cambridge, who gave me the benefit, early on in my research, of his extensive experience of the production of high quality petrography slides. Also R. Foley and M. Belatti of the Department of Biological Anthropology of the University of Cambridge. I. Chaplin of Buehler Krautkramer, to whom I am most grateful, aided the experimental work of best practice for sectioning teeth.

2. THE TECHNIQUE

OVERVIEW

The following steps, each of which is described in detail below, are involved in the production of a thin section:

1. Preparing the sample.
2. Removing the tooth from the jaw.
3. Encapsulating (or embedding) the sample in resin.
4. Cutting the section.
5. Grinding and polishing the section to ensure a flat surface suitable for bonding.
6. Bonding the section to a ground glass slide.
7. Cutting, grinding, and polishing the other side of the section to reduce it to 30 microns and bring to integrity.
8. Coverslipping.

In each of the above steps, meticulous care must be taken to ensure that the specimen is treated in a standard and therefore repeatable way that minimises potential damage to the cementum.

1) Sample Preparation

For any analysis to be meaningful, it is imperative that the samples are not exposed to any damage of the mineralised tissue. Therefore boiling and certainly bleaching in Sodium Perborate, standard methods of defleshing, are to be avoided. Burke & Castanet (1995) endorse the use of heated water and a solution of water and enzymes for defleshing. They refer to "thermal shock" occurring when the teeth are placed in boiling water and thus recommend that boiling water be avoided. In contrast, however, Crowe (1972) compared canines of Bobcats from the same skull placed in boiling water against canines prepared by maceration and found the numbers and intensity of the annuli in the teeth to be identical. To test these theories the author placed left side jaws from three Red deer into boiling water and three right sides from the same animal were defleshed using only immersion in cold water over a long period of time. Results indicated that the increments were slightly less clear on the teeth that had been boiled than those immersed in cold water, but the author could not identify "thermal shock".

An identical test was carried out to test the effects of bleaching and results show that this process makes it nearly impossible to distinguish between increments. Bleaching should therefore be avoided. However, the samples to be studied need to be dry and free from grease: if the specimen is wet or greasy, then the resin will not adhere to the surface or penetrate the sample. This can be quite difficult to achieve, especially for modern teeth, without the use of chemicals.

For modern specimens, the best method is to de-flesh them over a period of time by immersion in cold water (Grau, G.A., Sanderson, G.C.,Rogers J.P. 1970) changed daily, until most of the flesh and sinew has been removed by gentle rubbing of the bone between the index finger and thumb. They can then be left to dry at room temperature (Pike-Tay, pers. comm.). When the teeth are *completely* dry, they are ready to encapsulate. To dry throughout the teeth must be left for a week or more in dry conditions.

2) Removal of teeth from the jaw

Lieberman (1992) recommends that where possible, archaeological teeth are taken from jaws as cementum is likely to be stripped as a result of post-mortem processes, leading to false seasonal and age determinations. I support this recommendation fully.

Archaeologists have suggested that isolated teeth, or even pieces of teeth can be used (Spiess 1976, Beasley 1987, Beasley Brown & Legge 1992) and have even based the justification for destruction of the specimens on this assumption. However, as discussed in Chapter 1, cementum is a complex material that is still developing at death and would be susceptible to damage in the ground. As there already so many complications surrounding cementum incremental analysis, it would seem foolish to assume that any integrity could be obtained from isolated teeth and especially from small fragments of them.

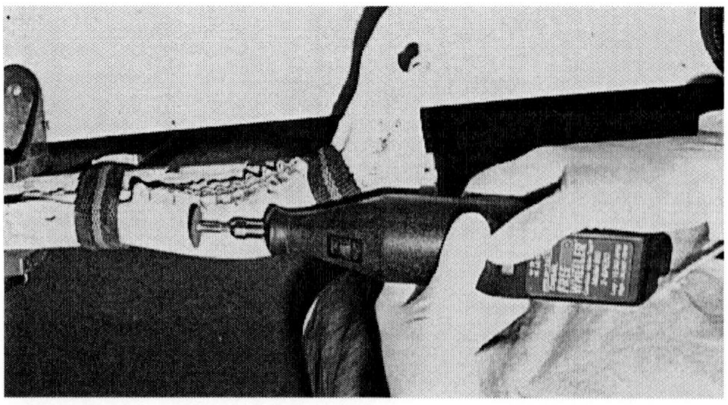

Figure 3 Removing a tooth from the jaw, using a Dremel saw. Photograph by Brown (1997)

For removal of teeth from the jaw, the following method was applied: a block of wood was secured in a vice. Hardwearing foam, about 3 cm thick, was secured onto the wood at either end of the jaw. The jaw was then held in place using standard luggage straps. In this way the jaw was held secure without damage to the bone or teeth. A window was then cut into the bone using a Dremel high-speed rotary saw (see Figure 3).

When the bone had been cut all the way around, the front of the bone was lifted off using a small screwdriver. Any bone around the apex of the root could be gently removed using a small sharp implement. The tooth was then gently levered out of the jaw. In this way the roots were untouched and therefore were not prone to damage.

2) Encapsulation

Encapsulation (also called embedding) of the tooth in resin serves to protect the sample, to produce a stable substance, and to assist handling. It is an essential component of the sectioning procedure. Archaeological material is often very brittle and therefore vulnerable to damage if it not encapsulated prior to sectioning. The resin needs to be as clear as possible so as not to interfere with analysis. Hillson (1986) used methyl methacrylate successfully for embedding archaeological material. I. Chaplin of Buehler tried this process on a number of the modern deer teeth from the collection of Red deer obtained for this thesis. The sections were exceptionally clear and well protected but the impregnation takes a number of weeks in controlled conditions and the resin is expensive and not as user friendly as some of the others used below.

Beasley, Brown & Legge (1992) examined various resins for encapsulation including two Buehler resins, Metset and "Epoxide", and Streuer's Epofix. They chose the latter for the embedding of archaeological teeth. Epoxy resins have a high shear strength and are quite colourless when hard (Humphries 1992).

There are two main methods of encapsulation, the principal difference between the two being the use of heat in setting:

1. Some resins, such as Petropoxy 154™ require heat to cure. Petropoxy is used in the production of geological and pottery thin sections (Ben Harris pers. comm. 1994). Lieberman (1992) advises against using resins which either require or produce heat, since they may make the tooth expand and crack. The author experimented with Petropoxy that requires heat added to cure, and experienced no difficulty with modern samples. Other resins were preferred on the grounds that Petropoxy is difficult to handle, and has a very pronounced yellow colour when set.

2. 'Cold' resins set after reaching an exothermic temperature, caused by a chemical reaction upon the mixing of the resin with the hardener. These resins do not require pressure or heat to cure.

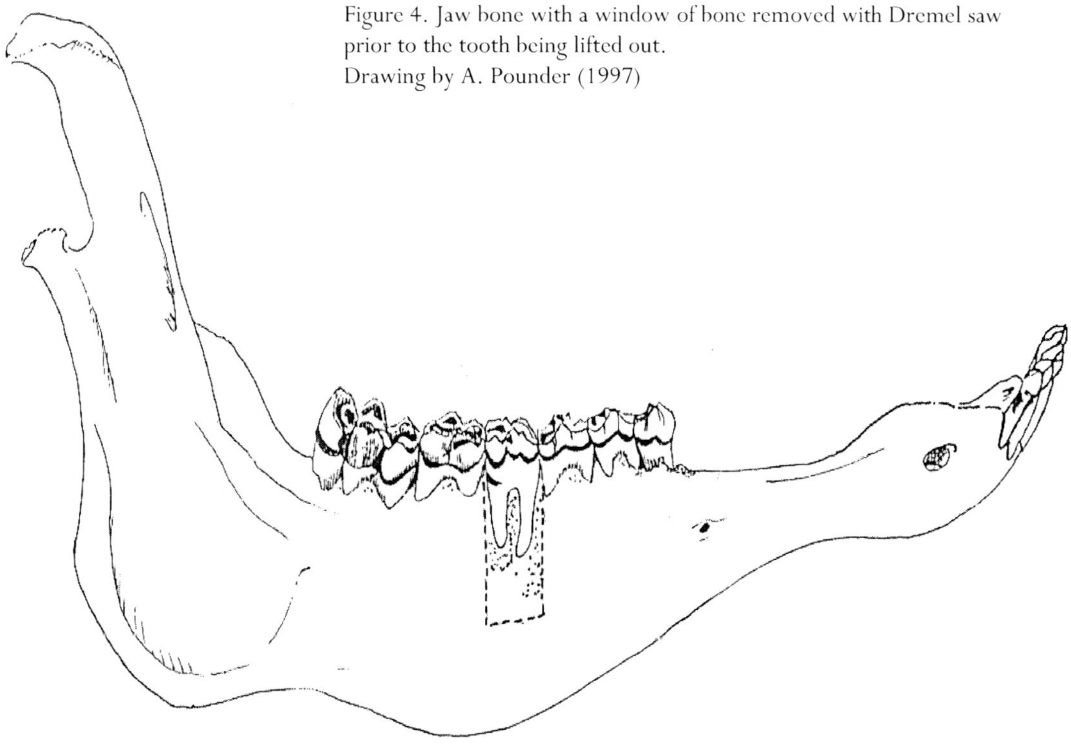

Figure 4. Jaw bone with a window of bone removed with Dremel saw prior to the tooth being lifted out.
Drawing by A. Pounder (1997)

It is very important that the resin adheres well to the sample, and does not contract. Care must be taken when mixing the resin and the hardener that bubbles are not added into the mixture. To ensure maximum penetration of the resin into the sample, the sample should be placed under vacuum as soon as the resin has been added: this drives air out of the sample, the resulting space being filled by resin. The sample is thus stabilised, reducing the possibility of loss or damage of the material during sectioning. The procedure employed was to hold the samples under vacuum for 15 minutes. The samples should then be left at room temperature until the resin has set completely (typically 8-12 hours).

Chaplin (pers.comm.) recommends pressure impregnation, and samples tried with this method were completely impregnated and very clear. However, a hole needs to be cut into the tooth to allow for complete impregnation and further equipment is needed, which was not practical for this research since the benefits were not sufficient to warrant the additional expenditure.[2]

Different resins have different consistencies, and as such take different amounts of time to set, to grind, and to polish. The first resin that used in this research was Buehler Epoxide™, which sets very hard and therefore presents an unacceptable contrast to the porosity and friability of the tooth, giving rise to setting problems within and in the immediate vicinity of the tooth. After rejecting Buehler Epoxide™, two different resins were used regularly:

1. **Buehler Epo-Thin Resin**™ This is a two-part mix of resin and hardener. Once mixed together, the two parts cause an exothermic reaction, at which point the mounted sample must be under vacuum. Epo-thin sets with a slight yellow tint, which becomes less obvious as the section becomes thinner. This tint, while not adversely affecting the interpretation of the section, is nevertheless difficult to ignore. Epo-Thin is a good all-purpose resin, which is a little cheaper than alternative resins in the same group.

2. **Epo-Tek 301**™ This is also a two part resin and hardener. While it has the advantage of setting clear, it is more sensitive that Epo-Thin to variations in room temperature and in the vacuum. Such variations give rise to bubbles in the resin that can obscure the outer edge of the tooth and can prevent the resin from adhering fully to the tooth.

Both of these resins set very hard: once hardened, they will remain so regardless of the conditions in which they are stored.

Encapsulation takes place in a small mounting cup, which, ideally, should be just a little larger than the tooth itself. If the cup is too large, then additional processing is

[2] Procedure for pressure impregnation.
Drill teeth to allow penetration of resin (0.5mm diameter). Vacuum the resin to remove dissolved gases (10-15 mins). Use a large beaker to allow room for frothing up. Vacuum range 76-100 centimetres. Place teeth in a moulding cup (tightly fitting and coated with release agent). Pour resin over teeth so that teeth are just covered by 2-3 mm of resin. Evacuate chamber, resin may froth up, allow air in and re-evacuate. Repeat 3-4 times. Finally leave under vacuum for 2 - 2 1/2 hours. Admit air and transfer to pressuring chamber at 2 bar and leave until resin is cured (minimum 8 hours).

Figure 5. If Burke's assumption is correct, bands and lines will be lost if the cut is not made through the centre of the tooth.

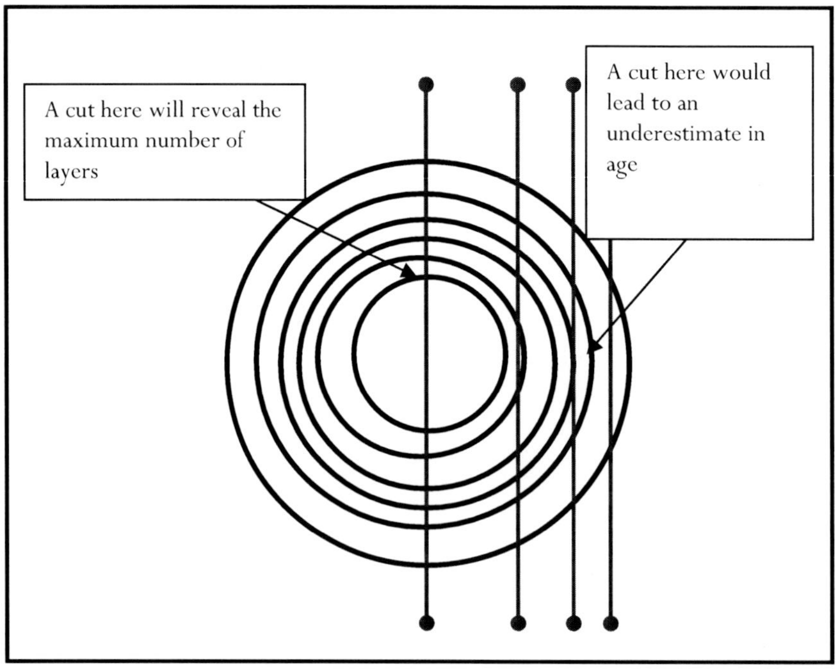

required in order to produce the thin section, due to the excess of resin involved; on the other hand, the sample should sit clear from the sides of the cup so that the whole sample is covered and held. A silicone release agent is applied to the mould before casting to aid with the removal of the cast specimen after the resin has hardened.

In this research, Buehler moulding cups were used: they have a loose bottom for ease of removal, and can be recycled.

4) Cutting the section

Once encapsulated, the tooth, within its resin block, is cut longitudinally through its centre from the crown to the root.

A Buehler Isomett ™ 1000 Diamond saw, equipped with a fixed diamond edged wheel, was used. This machine holds the specimen completely flat, while a diamond edged blade saws through it at a controlled speed (approximately 200 rpm). Both the type of blade used and the cutting speed are important: they affect both the quantity of the specimen that is lost, and the damage done to the remaining specimen.

The blade itself removes some of the specimen, and should therefore be as thin as possible in order to preserve as much of the sample as possible for further analysis. It is possible to use wafer-thin blades, provided that the resin is properly set, and the saw speed is not too fast. Various cutting wheels have been developed that use different types of abrasive, and it is important to be aware of the abrasiveness of the wheel chosen. Very abrasive blades not only remove much of the specimen, they also add damage to the specimen that needs to be removed by grinding and polishing. This, again, removes more of the sample than is necessary.

Burke (1992) suggests that, given the nature of cementum growth, it is very important to cut the section precisely in the centre of the tooth. Her assumption is that the cementum is laid down evenly, so that a number of increments may be lost if the cut is not made down the centre of the tooth. Omar (1992) took a number of sections from the same teeth of Red deer from Rum, and found that sections taken from the centre of the tooth showed the general pattern of bands, but that not every band extends to the edge of the cementum and that bands get narrower at the edge of the specimens.

After cutting, and after each stage of grinding and polishing, the sample should ideally be examined under reflected light at a magnification of x100. There are two reasons for doing this:

1. To ensure that damage to the sample is progressively being removed, and no extra damage is created.

2. To make records of the material before it is removed at each step. In this way, it is possible to observe how the cementum varies at different levels of the tooth: most researchers only study a single slice through the tooth. In this way the importance of cutting through the centre of the tooth can be assessed.

Figure 6. The cut must be made through the centre of the tooth. Figure after Hillson 1986

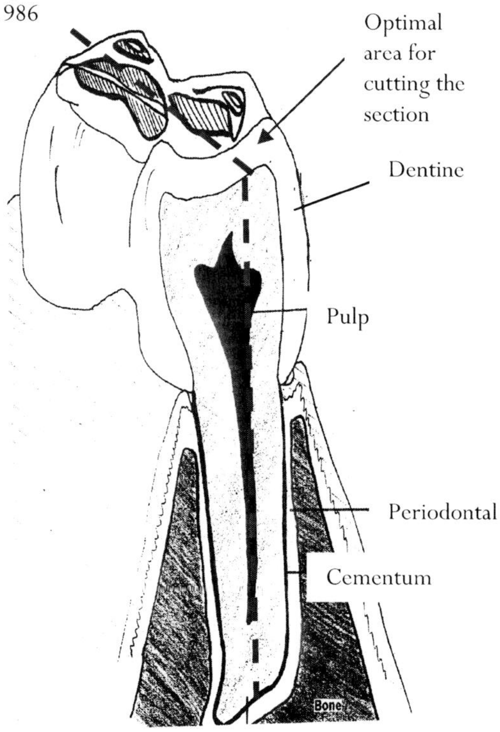

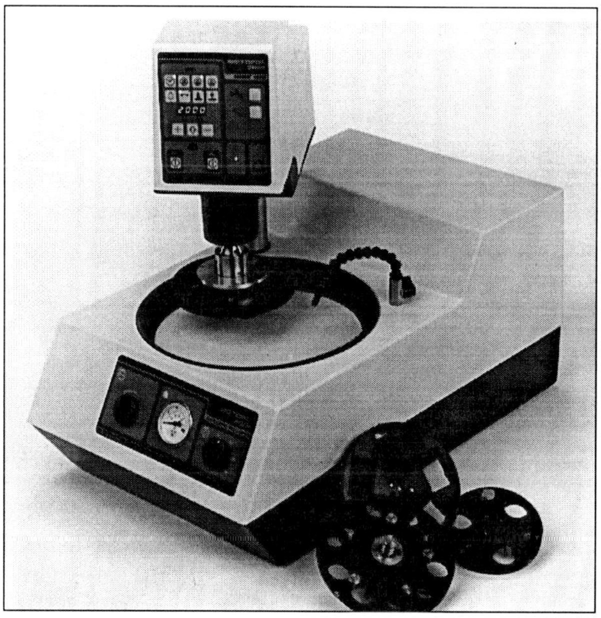

Figure 7. The Buehler Motopol™
Photograph courtesy of Buehler Krautkramer Ltd.

5) Grinding and Polishing the Section

Either or both of the two halves of the tooth can be used to produce thin sections: if one half is not used, then it can be preserved for future research. The half that is to be made into a thin section must be ground and polished to bring it to integrity and to ensure that it will bond with a glass slide.

1. **Grinding** is the process of removing damage (scratches caused by the cutting wheel) on the surface of the sample, the aim being to make the section completely flat prior to bonding. It is distinct from lapping, a technique used by geologists in the production of petrographical thin sections. Lapping involves the use of loose abrasives, while grinding involves the use of fixed abrasives: loose abrasives cause less shock to the sample, but can dirty it and are less efficient at speed. They work by having slurries of powdered abrasive suspended in water or oil and spread over a glass or cast iron plate (Hillson 1986).

Each grinding stage removes a little more damage, but is itself an aggressive process; thus it is necessary to gradually decrease the abrasive size to decrease the level of damage on the surface. Various grades of Silicon Carbide paper were used for grinding, from 600 - p2500 grit. These were stuck onto a 12" diameter aluminium platen that is mechanically rotated using the Buehler Motopol™. This machine allows for six sections to be processed simultaneously by holding them in a specially made specimen holder that is lowered onto the rotating platen at a desired pressure. This machine ensures that a clean and flat surface, free of pits, hollows and scratches is achieved.

The sections are clamped into a holder, and lowered onto the Silicon Carbide paper on top of a rotating platen. The grind is uniform since the specimen is driven in a complementary direction to the platen: such uniformity would be very difficult (and time-consuming) to achieve by hand grinding. The Motopol allows for complete control over the pressure applied to the samples on the paper, the speed of the platen and the amount of lubricant being used. The coarse paper is used to begin with to remove bulk quickly. The grinding is to remove the damage put into the specimen by the cutting process, so the less aggressive the cut, the less material need be wasted in the grinding process. "A knowledge of how the material removal occurs and the subsequent damage resulting from this working is vital to our knowledge if progressing the surface to integrity is to be achieved." (Buehler work manual 1994). Water is used as a lubricant in the grinding process, and it is important to carefully control the flow of this. If there is too little water, the sample will be greatly damaged by burning or rubbing against the carbide; while if there is too much water, then a film is produced which the specimen has to work against, and this also produces a poor quality section.

In general, the process used on taking sections from the saw was as follows: after each of the steps below, the sample was washed in water, dried, and rinsed in acetone.

1. Grind for 3 minutes at p600 grit Silicon Carbide (average grit size 16 μm).
2. Grind for 5 minutes at 800 grit (average grit size 12 μm).

3. Grind for 5 minutes at 1200 grit (average grit size 6.5 µm).[3]
4. Polish

2. **Polishing** Once a perfect grind has been achieved and most of the damage has been removed, the sections are polished. Polishing removes the final scratches, which results in the section having a shine on the surface. This is achieved using diamond pastes. The diamond paste is added to a cloth with a dense nap surface. This nap cloth sits on a platen for use with the Motopol. To polish, rather than scratch or grind, a lubricant is added. The lubricant used in this case was a Collodial Silica polishing suspension, a non-scratching abrasive.

Various grades of diamond paste, beginning with 10 micron diamond and ending with 3 micron diamond are used. As with the grinding process above, the section is cleaned between each change of paste using acetone.

Caution is necessary at this stage, since over-polishing results in smearing of the surface, loss of integrity, and even a little peeling of the surface. To avoid this, the polishing should be performed carefully and slowly, with just the right amount of lubricant and with very little pressure. After polishing the surface is completely flat, clear and free of scratches caused by sawing and grinding.

6) Bonding the section

Once the section has been ground and polished, it is ready to be bonded (mounted) to a glass slide. For maximum clarity, the slide should be as thin as possible. It should, however be thick enough to sustain the bulk of a deer molar in resin.

The glass slide should be ground flat before any bonding is attempted: this also gives relief, which ensures a stronger bond between the slide and the mounted specimen.

Both the glass slide and the specimen need to be clean and free from grease. "The principal requirements of a mounting medium are strong adhesion to the glass, long term stability and a high refractive index" (Humphries 1992).

There are two good choices of bonding medium: either the same resin that was used for encapsulation, or a photocement such as Norland Optical Adhesive 61 (which produces more rapid results).

1. **Use of the encapsulation resin:** The resin is mixed and applied to the slide. The section is placed on top, and gently manoeuvred until no air remains between the section and the slide (any remaining air weakens the bond and distorts observation). The section must then be placed on a bonding gig until the resin has hardened, in order to ensure a strong zero bond (i.e. with nothing between the section and the slide). The resin typically takes 8-12 hours to harden.

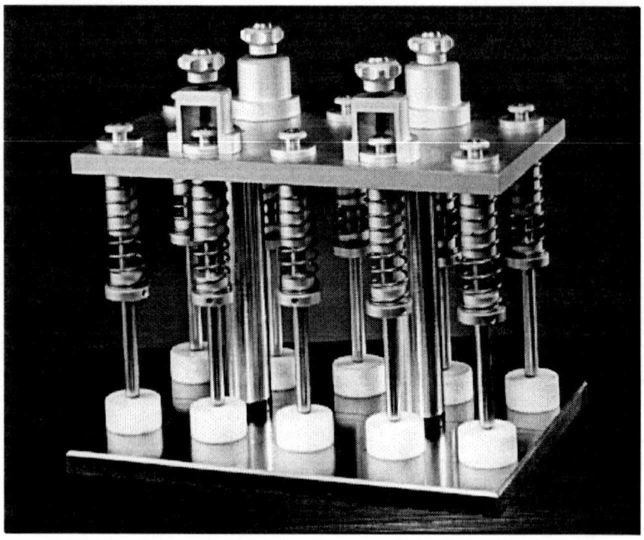

Figure 8. The Bonding Jig.
Photograph courtesy of Buehler Krautkramer Ltd.

2. **Use of photocements:** A photocement is a glue which hardens quickly when it is exposed to UV light (sun or artificial). It sets much more quickly than epoxy resins (typically in 10-30 minutes, although a longer setting time may improve the bond), and is also easier to manipulate, since it does not begin to set until exposed to UV light. A bonding gig is required for an ideal bond. Though Humphries (1992) recommends that photocements are not used for bonding, the sections in this thesis that were bonded using Norland Optical Adhesive 61 were highly successful. The bond was strong and clear and the adhesive easy to use. The speed of setting meant that it was much less susceptible to heat, moisture and humidity which adversely affected the bonding of sections using epoxy resin.

To avoid contamination, the technique described above requires that the working environment be clean, and maintained at a constant temperature and humidity. While hardening, the resin is affected adversely by changes in temperature, and it will not harden clear if the room is too humid. These requirements can be problematic if working in a shared laboratory.

7) Final reduction of the section

Once the section has been bonded, it is necessary to remove the top bulk in order to reduce the section to 30 microns, the optimum thickness for observing

[3] European grit numbers are different from those used in the U.S.A. To avoid confusion when using European sizes the letter "P" is placed before the grit numbers. (Buehler workbook 1994)

increments. There are three ways to do this: the choice of method depends on a) whether or not it is desirable to preserve as much as possible of the specimen; b) the friability of the specimen; and c) the required speed of production.

1. **Using the Buehler Petrothin™ (following Lieberman 1992):** This method has the advantage of being very fast. The Petrothin has a diamond blade (using which the bulk section can be cut from the slide), and a fixed high speed diamond grinding disc to grind down the remaining section. Although it is fast, this method results in the loss of a great deal of the sample: the fixed diamond is 100 microns, and therefore quite abrasive, and the Petrothin saw is also quite thick, thus removing up to 3 mm of the specimen. Lieberman advises examination of the specimen directly from the Petrothin. I found this method adequate, although the specimen was somewhat damaged: it is better to repeat the procedure of grinding and polishing outlined above once the sample has come off the Petrothin, in order to bring the section to integrity for effective analysis.
2. **Grinding to integrity without cutting off the bulk first:** If the section is already quite thin, then it can be ground without the need to cut off the bulk first. This can be done either by hand, or on the Motopol using a holder.

3. **Cutting using the Isomett thin diamond blade:** For best results, the bulk should be cut off the sample using the Isomett ™ saw with a thin diamond blade. Having cut very close to the slide, grinding and polishing to the required thickness can be carried out with minimal destruction. Using this method, it is possible to obtain 5 or 6 sections from a single tooth if required, whereas the maximum possible using the Petrothin is only 4.

8) Coverslipping

Coverslipping protects the finished section. Excess resin is removed from around the section using a razor blade. As with the mounting, the resin used for embedding and/or mounting can be used to adhere the coverslip to the section. Norland Optical Adhesive was the preferred option as it is very easy to handle and did not need excessive pressure to remove the air bubbles between the coverslip and the section. The coverslip is first cleaned with acetone and a small amount of adhesive is added before the coverslip is carefully lowered onto the section. Gentle pressure is then applied to the coverslip to force the air out.

Chapter Four
Incremental analysis of a modern control sample of Red deer

1. BACKGROUND

The initial aim of this research was to establish the optimal method for estimating the absolute age and season of death of Red deer using cementum incremental analysis, and to determine the accuracy and reliability of the technique. Decalcification was not considered appropriate as it cannot be used on archaeological teeth. Spiess (1979) was only able to use 10 out of 171 thin sections of archaeological teeth after decalcification (see Chapter 3). The decision was therefore made to examine standard ground thin sections. It was intended that one of the principal ways that this research would improve upon earlier work was that all of the experiments would be based on a large modern control sample, including many of known age and date of death. It was proposed that, once the technique had been developed and all of the discrepancies noted by other authors had been investigated, the technique should be applied to archaeological Red deer in order to establish the season of occupation of archaeological sites. As has already been mentioned, other researchers have experienced substantial difficulties in assembling modern collections on which such an analysis can be based (see for example Pike-Tay 1991). Pike-Tay (1995) examined a large modern population of 677 Caribou teeth. However, she does not make it clear how many of the sample were known aged (tagged at birth) and how many were aged using tooth wear and previous cementum analysis; nor does she specify how many of the sections she produced herself and how many had been made previously. Hitherto, the only study of incremental analysis based upon a large modern population of 113 known aged (tagged at birth) Red deer that was carried out using standard ground thin sections is that of Omar (1992).

2. COLLECTION AND DESCRIPTION OF THE MODERN POPULATION SAMPLE

Method of collection and acknowledgements

My first approach was to Professor Clutton Brock of the Department of Zoology of the University of Cambridge, who has worked with Red deer for many years and heads up the most extensive study of Red deer ever undertaken, on the Scottish Island of Rum. With his support I was able to get in touch with many gamekeepers and wildlife managers, with the British Deer Society and with the Deer Commission for Scotland. I also approached Mrs. Norma Chapman, an acknowledged authority on deer whom I knew to be in possession of known aged populations of both Red and Fallow deer.

I am very grateful to a number of people without whose assistance my collection of modern material would not have been possible. In particular, I am indebted to Hugh Rose of the British Deer Society and to Colin McLean of the Deer Commission for Scotland (formerly the Red Deer Commission): they enabled me to collect jaws from a number of estates, including Euston, Balmoral, Wormsley Park, Abernethy, and Wollaton Park. I am also grateful to all the gamekeepers and park rangers who obtained and saved jaws for me, including Des Dugan, J Mayfield, Mr. Pall, Peter Ord, and Sandy Masson. Colin McLean of the Deer Commission for Scotland supplied a large number of Red deer mandibles of known age whose dates of death covered every month of the year, a seemingly unique basis from which to undertake a study of incremental analysis.

The Sample

All jaws collected were lower mandibles with complete dentition, including the incisors. The collection was started with around 40 jaws from Euston in Suffolk, which had been shot during the English hunting season. They were kindly donated by Hugh Rose. Subsequently, a large number of jaws was obtained from the Deer Commission for Scotland: all were of known date of death, but of unknown age. These came from Ben Arnine, Srath Vaich, Achentoul, Lynaberack, Creag Meagadih, and Glen Doe – see the table below for the number of jaws from each estate. These estates are scattered across Scotland, and represent a wide range of different environments. Most of the jaws were from stags shot between August and October, except for the Ben Arnine collection, which comprised males shot between August and October, and females shot between October and February. All of the animals concerned had been aged by experienced stalkers and gamekeepers, using tooth wear and body weight and condition. These age estimates were not taken into consideration until the teeth had been sectioned and the analysis completed.

In addition, I was supplied with a very valuable sample comprising 91 jaws of known age, coming from animals which had been tagged at birth and were of known date of death. They were collected over a long period of time, and included a full range of ages from 5 months to 16 years. They came from a variety of locations in the Scottish Highlands.
Additional jaws from Scottish Red deer were obtained from Abernethy and from Balmoral. The Abernethy collection comprised 43 males and 13 females of known date of death but unknown age, which covered December, January, February, and October. The Balmoral collection comprised both sides of 12 jaws, which enabled me to make a comparison of the results of all techniques when applied to different sides of the same jaw. There were no noticeable differences between the two sides of the jaw, either for incremental analysis or for ageing by wear. Both sides of the jaw are therefore

appropriate for these techniques for Red deer.[1] These animals were all from the same herd, and were killed simultaneously by an avalanche. Because their death was accidental, the animals encompassed a broad age range, and there was an approximately equal number of each sex.

Jaws collected from locations in England included 17 from Wormsley Deer Park, which all died on the same day; and 10 from Wollaton in Nottingham, of known date of death but unknown age.

The following table provides a summary of the modern collection. A total of 230 successful thin sections were initially created from this sample; 770 sections were unsuccessful. A variety of difficulties that can give rise to unsuccessful sections are described later in this chapter.

	Number of Animals			Age and Date of Death	
Location	Male	Female	Unknown Sex	Known Age	Known Date
Euston	35	6		No	Yes
Ben Arnine	40	25	70	No	Yes
Srath Vaich	70			No	Yes
Achentoul	73			No	Yes
Lynaberack	50			No	Yes
Creag Meagadih	27			No	Yes
Glen Doe	70			No	Yes
Highlands	26	41	24	Yes	Yes
Abernethy	43	13		No	Yes
Balmoral			12	No	Yes
Wormsley			17	No	Yes
Wollaton			10	No	Yes

Table 4: Provenance of modern control collection.

In addition, Colin McLean supplied me with a sample of 15 Sika deer calves and yearlings, dating from October to June. These were also sectioned, and it was found that there were no substantial differences in analysis between Red deer and Sika deer. Figure 9 shows a 50 micron Sika thin section. The dark area indicated in the the picture is dentine, directly above which sits the neonatal line. 4 bands can be counted, one of which is darker in colour than the others. There are also between 5 and 6 thinner black lines, normally interpreted as "winter" lines, in this area. The outer edge is a dark line, suggesting (correctly for this animal) a winter death. The very light material which adheres to the edge of the tooth is tissue.

A choice had to be made as to which teeth should be sectioned first when the sectioning technique was still being developed. The first sections were from teeth of unknown age from the larger Scottish and English samples (Ben Arnine and Euston). Once the technique had been fully established, the last teeth to be sectioned were from the sample of known age and date of death. However, not all of this sample was sectioned: this was a decision taken by the author, who was by this time convinced that cementum incremental analysis is deeply

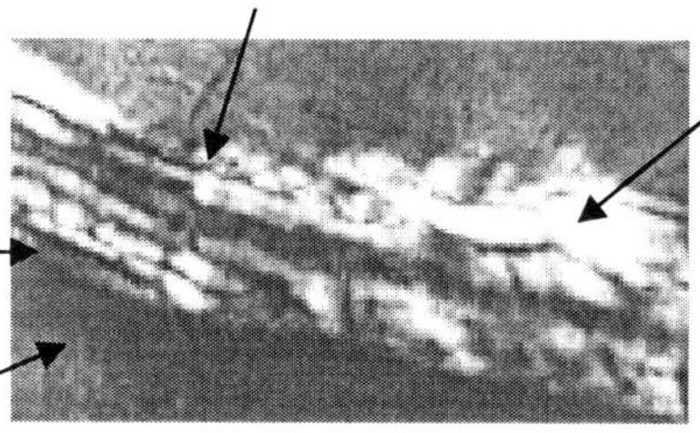

Figure 9. Section of Sika deer tooth

flawed, and did not wish to damage the remainder of the sample. However, in order to carry out the broadest possible analysis, one section from each year group was prepared, and these were chosen in an attempt to cover the widest possible range of seasons. All of the jaws were also examined using a new scoring scheme (see Chapters 5 and 6).

The importance of using a control population which is as close as possible to the archaeological population being studied has been stressed (Burke 1992). This would be the ideal, but as has already been explained, it is difficult to obtain any modern population of known age and date of death, even when no attempt is made to match the environment, diet, and species with a given archaeological population. Even if all of these factors could be matched, the sample could still not be used as a "catch all" group, since of course different archaeological sites cover different time periods and provide broadly different environments. Additionally, modern control samples are required for all species being studied. Pike-Tay (1996) points out that only by studying a large modern population can many of the problems associated with thin section interpretation be overcome species by species.

The modern jaws obtained for researching the issues in this study were from a wide variety of environments. From the start, there was no single archaeological site to which it was envisaged the technique would be applied, and therefore there was no need to attempt to match environments. Environmental differences from which the animals were obtained were recorded when the thin sections were analysed and when tooth wear analysis was being carried out in this study.

3. TECHNIQUE OF ANALYSIS

Entering into the field of incremental analysis without previous experience, it was necessary for me to base my analysis on previous research. I began by finding out how to create a thin section, and in particular how to create a thin section of a tooth. I was very fortunate to be aided by Dr. Robert Foley and Margaret Belattie of the Department of Anthropology of the University of Cambridge, who both had experience of tooth thin sectioning.

Foley warned me that preparation techniques can damage cementum and, when a tooth is being sectioned for the

[1] This may not be the case for all species, as Foley (1986) in his study of tropical ungulates found that left and right M1s of the same animal may have different cementum layer counts.

purpose of cementum analysis, it is advisable to check at every stage that the cementum is intact and has not been damaged by the preparation process. This was taken into consideration, and tested on several jaws of unknown age. The value of Foley's observation soon became apparent: many preparation techniques can make incremental analysis impossible as they damage the cementum.

Preparation of the Jaws

Initially, a selection of jaws was prepared by the standard defleshing route used to clean bones for comparative collections. This process begins by boiling the jaws in stocking cloth (in case the teeth fall out) for about two hours. The jaws are then placed in Sodium Perborate, which essentially bleaches the bone. Although this system is appropriate for the cleaning of bones and jaws for teaching collections, it was soon discovered that it makes the reading of cementum increments impossible. The teeth became white coloured, and the cementum layers became indiscernible. Ignorance was the key factor involved: in particular, the author's lack of understanding of cementum as a mineralised tissue. Klevezal (1996) notes that when material has been bleached by Hydrogen Peroxide, it is very difficult to distinguish layers as the bleaching destroys marginal layers of bone. In cattle teeth that had been bleached, Klevezal noticed a white surface over the whole tooth, including the outer layer of cementum; she also observed that the layers of these teeth were poorly stained. She remarked that strong detergents would have the same effect. Although preparation techniques and storage are essential elements of incremental analysis, very few authors include details of the preparation techniques undertaken prior to sectioning in their reports.

Subsequently, all jaws were soaked in cold water which was changed daily, and the flesh was removed carefully by gentle rubbing, as recommended by Pike-Tay (1996 pers. comm.). This ensured preservation of the cementum. Further details of this defleshing process are given in Chapter 3.

Thin section production and associated problems

The production of thin sections is described in detail in Chapter 3. In presenting a more historical account of the development of the technique, and in order to describe some of the pitfalls that can arise, it is worth noting that problems encountered in the production of these thin sections were many and varied. At first there were severe problems in getting the resin to adhere to the teeth. This left a gap between the tooth and the resin. A gap would prevent the resin from protecting the tooth during thin section production. Not only could the section be damaged, but interpretation could become misleading, not only as a result of the damage, but also as a result of misinterpreting the light at the edge of the tooth. The solution was to degrease the teeth by cleaning with acetone before impregnation. It was also found that impregnation without a vacuum was unacceptable, as the specimen would not adhere fully to the tooth, even if it had been previously degreased. The vacuum is required to ensure that all the air surrounding the tooth is removed.

In order to establish the optimal use of the vacuum pump, a number of experiments were carried out. A sample of specimens were cut in half, with one half being vacuum impregnated and the other half being left to harden without the use of the vacuum. Having established that vacuum impregnation was necessary, further experiments were carried out to establish the optimum amount of time required to vacuum: enough to ensure that all of the air is removed, but not so much as to create an accelerated curing of the resin that would result in bubbles. It was found that the optimal impregnation time was 20 minutes.

Impregnation of teeth is vital in order to protect the outer incremental layers during sectioning. Clevedon, Brown and Hilton (1979) noted that a histological section is itself an artefact, and that the processes of the living cells are arrested, the protein structure precipitated, and many labile substances lost. However, as can be seen in Figure 10, if the tooth is weak in any area then forcing epoxy into the tooth can damage it. Often "artefacts" occur during fixation or sectioning: the differential hardness or rigidity of different tissue constituents, when subjected to dehydration and embedding processes, may result in splits in the tissue and other distortions which need to be recognised (Clevedon, Brown and Hilton 1979). The tooth shown in Figure 10 was clearly weak, and the epoxy filled the gap that was caused by the tooth cracking. This is a modern tooth which was prepared with maximum care: the chances of such a tooth being able to survive in the ground for thousands of years, and then to be sectioned successfully for age or seasonality determination are extremely remote.

Figure 10. Tooth split as resin embedded

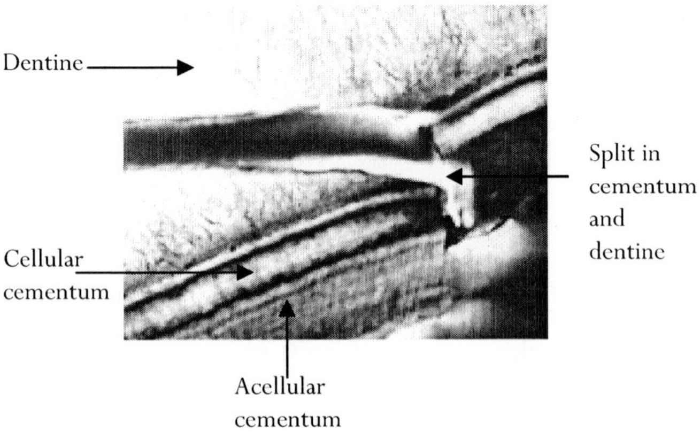

Another problem which arose was lifting of the sample. This can occur if the resin is exposed to excess humidity or to temperature variations which prevent it from setting properly. This not only leaves a region of the tooth insufficiently protected against the sectioning technique, but can also mean that the sample is not properly adhered to the glass slide, so that it lifts and cannot be studied accurately. As Clevedon, Brown and Hilton (1979) note, such accidents in the production of thin sections can lead to misinterpretation of the data, and "folding or buckling of the sections can be misleading to the uninitiated."

Difficulties in interpretation can also arise if the thin section is not exactly flat, because the incremental layers are light sensitive. A section which has been improperly made in this way could have a shadow around its edge, which might well be mistaken for a 'dark layer'.

Ben Harris of the Department of Geology of the University of Cambridge provided essential experience in the production of thin sections. Geological thin sections are made in a very similar way to the standard ground thin sections used in incremental analysis. It was with the help of Harris that the author was able to test different impregnation and grinding techniques. Generally the blades needed to cut thin sections of rock are much too abrasive for teeth. Geological thin sections are ground using wet silicon carbide on a lapping wheel. This was found to make the section very dirty and was therefore unsuitable for teeth. I was also helped by Rod Long of the Department of Geology of the University of Cambridge, who taught me how to make casts of teeth prior to sectioning. A cast was produced of all the known aged teeth prior to sectioning. Casting of teeth, particularly arcaheological teeth, is essential to preserve information on crown height and other measurements. A good cast can also be used to replace teeth from jaws in museum collections.

As outlined in Chapter 3, it was decided that it would be futile to develop a thin sectioning technique for the modern control sample which couldn't thereafter be applied to archaeological material. Given the numerous problems with cementum incremental analysis, it would be absurd to add further complication by using two very different methods of thin sectioning.

Having decided that production of a thin section using standard ground techniques was advisable, and after much discussion with people experienced in the production of thin sections, this method was perfected (see Chapter 3). The initial cut was always made longitudinally through the centre of the tooth, and one half of the tooth (always the buccal side) was kept as a "thick section": that is, half a tooth held in resin with the cementum visible. After the first cut the tooth is separated into two thick sections, both of which can be examined for incremental layers using reflected light microscopy.

Initially the Buehler Isomet 100™ low speed saw was used for cutting the sections. However, this was found to be very slow, and this hindered the rapid production of thin sections. Moreover, grinding through to the slide lost a lot of material. The saw was therefore upgraded to a larger Buehler Isomet 1000™ so that the slides could be cut at regular intervals, thus protecting as much of the material as possible.
After the initial cut, the lingual side was then cut again and ground to make the thin section. It was essential that these cuts were made in exactly the same way for every tooth, and that the same side of the tooth was viewed in every section. Similarly, it was imperative to position all of the teeth on the slide in the same way. Thus any differences in cementum deposition which became apparent under analysis were the result of the cementum structure itself, and not of the sectioning technique or of the section orientation.

4. EXAMINATION TECHNIQUE

In general, both thick sections and thin sections of all teeth were examined. The sectioning technique is described in detail in Chapter 3. Using a technique where the section is gradually taken down allows for examination of the cementum at varying thickness, thus enabling constant checks on any damage that may have been caused to the cementum.

Examination of standard ground thin sections of a modern control sample of Red deer

A wide variety of potential problems with sectioning technique have already been described. Assuming that the technique has been perfected, that the samples are not contaminated in any way, and that the microscopical technique is equally well understood, then incremental analysis should in principal be a straightforward process. There are difficulties in interpreting the material and, as explained in Chapter 1, an understanding of the different types of cementum is vital. The following discussion, therefore, is based upon the assumption that all possible care had been taken to ensure accurate interpretation of the sections, and that any discrepancies in the material are a result of the tissue itself rather than of the sectioning process. Some of the issues which this research was attempting to address are listed below:

1. The reliability of cementum incremental analysis: that is, the extent to which a single observer, or two different observers, can reliably obtain the same readings from the same section.
2. The optimal area of the tooth to examine for age and seasonality assessment.
3. Whether or not cementum deposition varied around the tooth.
4. Whether or not seasonality estimation was consistent over the surface of a single tooth, and between teeth.
5. Whether secondary increments were consistent, and if not whether they were more likely to appear in certain locations on the tooth.

To this end, all of the sections were examined meticulously several times, and the results of the examinations were recorded on the sheet reproduced in Appendix 2. This sheet also identfies the various locations A, B, C, D, E, F, G, H, X, Y, and Z around the tooth at which measurements were made, and which are referred to in the following discussion.

It should be remarked at this point that the reliability of cementum incremental analysis is very poor, as demonstrated later on in this chapter. That is to say, even a single observer cannot reliably replicate his measurements on a given section. This degree of subjectivity in the analysis should be taken into account when considering the results given below. Other authors have also noted that the subjectivity of layer counts is one of the main disadvantages of ageing by means of cementum incremental analysis (Smirnov 1983, 1984, Klevezal 1996). As cementum incremental analysis can be subjective, the interpretations of the sections discussed in this study are those of the author.

When faced with a jaw, or even an isolated tooth, for incremental analysis, it would be easy for a researcher familiar with tooth development to hazard a guess at the age of the animal, even if that age is unknown. Broadly speaking, the pulp cavity is wide and open in young animals, is part filled when the animal is approximately five years old, and can be full by the time the animal is over seven years old. Nearly all of the literature on incremental analysis claims that the accuracy of the results is based upon incremental analysis alone: it is, however, impossible to say, given the subjectivity of counting layers, how much the researchers' readings have been subconsciously influenced by this obvious marker of age. Every attempt was made here to ignore this marker, and to base the results on incremental analysis alone.

For the purposes of this study I will demonstrate the type of observations made, and the potential difficulties which can arise in making such observations, using the sample of known age and date of death animals. All of these sections were meticulously prepared once the sectioning technique had been perfected, all were first molars, and all were examined using the same microscope under the same conditions. They were examined under polarised transmitted light at magnifications of X100 and X40.

All of the jaws in the sample were from Red deer, which calve between May and June (Clutton Brock et al 1982) each year. The seasons of death of the animals can therefore be obtained from their known ages.

An additional area was considered for this section, between locations D and Y (see Figure 11). At this one location alone, two bands and one line can be seen, with a supplementary band of cellular cementum which can be seen very clearly in Figure 13. At an area very close to this point, Figure 12 shows a bright neo-natal line, a thick dark band, and then two bands and two lines. On the remainder of the section, either one or two each of bands and lines could be discerned. Another noteworthy point concerning this section is that the bands at location X are particularly clear, but that there is a definite merging of the dentine on the dentine/cementum junction. The layers were clear and straight, and there was a clear neo-natal line (which inexperienced observers might interpret as an incremental layer). The section had a light outer edge, which would suggest a summer or very early winter death. If only the area shown in Figure 12 were analysed, there would be accurate assumptions about age and season of death, as the last band is very wide and would suggest an end of summer death. The important point is that the cementum is not consistent around this tooth, and though it is easy to convince oneself of accuracy when the age is known, it would be difficult without prior knowledge to say which location should provide an accurate assessment of age and season of death.

Specimen 1: 1 year 7 months, Male. Died December / January

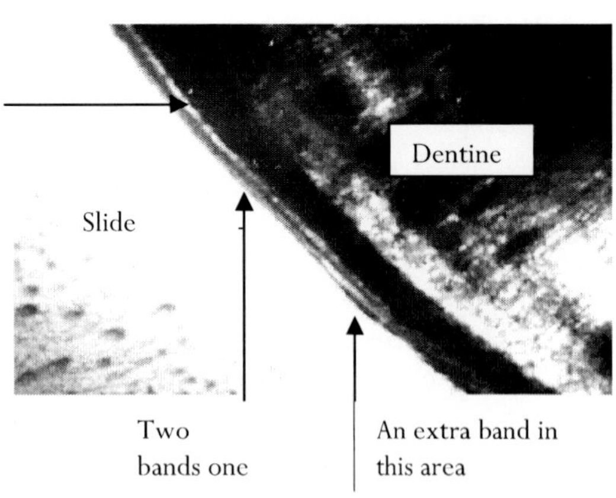

Figure 11. Mag X40 between D and Y

Figure 12

Mag X100

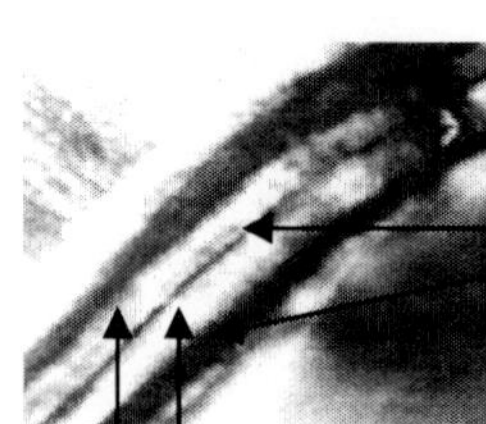

Figure 13

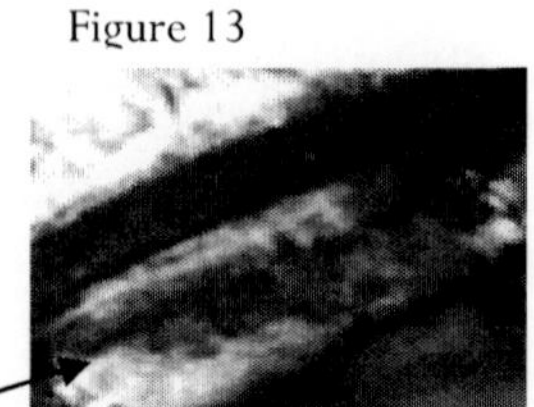

Summary

Any observer would conclude that this section came from an animal that was certainly over two years old, and perhaps three years old, depending on the area of the tooth which was studied. If the whole of the section was examined, it would be tempting to age the animal by the maximum number of bands and lines which could be seen, leading to an age estimation of three years or greater. If the observer were familiar with tooth development, then it would be obvious from the pulp cavity that the animal could not be this old, and some conscious or subconscious adjustment might be made. Given the inaccuracy of the age estimation, it is hardly surprising that seasonality cannot be accurately assessed.

Specimen 2: 2years 8 months, Male, Died January / February.

Location H showed a single thick band of cellular cementum, which seems to indicate that some resorption has taken place. This may be the result of injury, or of unusual stress placed upon the tooth. The animal is young enough that it seems unlikely to have been caused by movement through the jaw. A good deal of damage was also apparent at location A, with no 'readable' layers visible.

At location F there are up to five bands and five lines visible, with a small area of cellular cementum overlaying the acellular cementum: this again would suggest some resorption, or a need to fill a gap between the cementum and the bone. This is consistent with the evidence of damage or movement on the other side of the section. The lines are not as clearly defined as in other sections. The cause of this is not understood, but it may have something to do with the speed at which cementum is being deposited (Berkovitz et al 1995).

Figure 14.

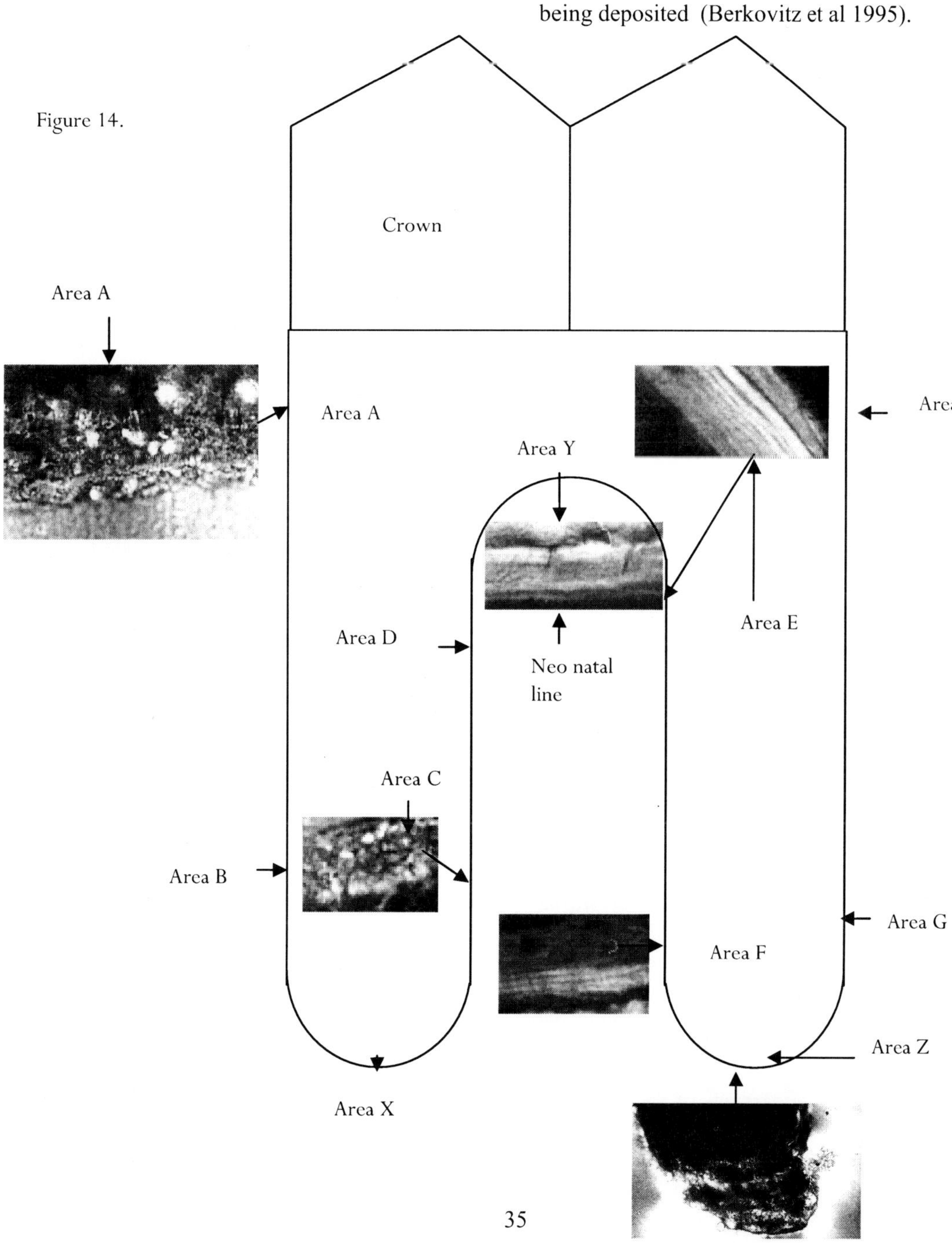

Location E was particularly clear, showing four bands and four lines. The outer layer is clearly a line, which would be interpreted (correctly) as a winter death. The total number of discernible bands and lines varies around the tooth from a single line to five bands and five lines. The photograph at this location shows the neo-natal line beside the dentine. As with specimen 1, an inexperienced observer might be led to interpret this as adding to the age of the animal, since bands and lines can be seen within the neo-natal line. It is clear from this photograph that more bands and lines exist than are consistent with a single band and a single line being laid down each year. Also, this single photograph demonstrates a transition from a dark to a light outer layer. The cementum at location C is very pitted, and shows severe areas of damage, and regions of cellular cementum. The tubules in the dentine can be seen very clearly. It would be impossible to estimate age or season of death from this location. The pad cementum (location Y) doesn't show the number of bands and lines one would expect in an animal this age. In location G there are two quite clear lines and bands, with a dark outer layer suggesting a winter death. An observer who studied this one location would therefore make an accurate assessment of age and season of death.

Summary

It is clear from this tooth just how variable the incremental structure can be in different locations on the tooth.

If only a single location were examined on this tooth, it would most probably be either A or H, since most of the literature claims that these locations are the clearest and easiest to interpret. However location A has been completely altered and is not suitable for incremental analysis. It is clear from the other locations that no single assessment of age or seasonality could be made from a thorough study of this tooth, even though it is a modern sample which was prepared as precisely as possible. It might be argued in some cases that different microscopical techniques and additional experience in microscopy might lead to an improved assessment: however, this tooth is evidently unusable for incremental analysis, regardless of the microscopical technique that is used.

Specimen 3: 3 years 7 months, Female, Died December / January

The outer layer of this section varied in thickness around the tooth, and could give rise to a seasonality assessment of late winter/early summer (location E), end of winter (locations C, D, and G), or beginning of winter (locations A and B). Clearly if such a tooth, or a fragment of it, were found on an archaeological site, this discrepancy (compounded by the other issues associated with archaeological material) would make it extremely unlikely that an accurate assessment of the season of occupation of the site could be made.

In location Y, the outer lacunae band showed ridging and banding similar to that seen in acellular cementum, with at least six bands and lines present. At location H the layer closest to the dentine was split in two, with up to five split or false increments between H and G.
Between locations C and D the tooth root was misshapen, with a distinct curve.

Specimen 4: 4 years 5 months, Female, Died October / November

The root edge is very light in this section, due to a lack of dense mineralisation, and has very broad lacunae. The greatest number of bands and lines visible at any location is two, in locations A, G, and H. The accompanying photograph (Figure 15) clearly shows two broad bands and two thin lines, which split and bifurcate to give four bands and four lines. The outer edge remains dark, which could be the result of tissue adhering or of the microscopical technique, since this edge is unnaturally thick. The outermost layer was dark in most locations, correctly suggesting a winter death.

Figure 15

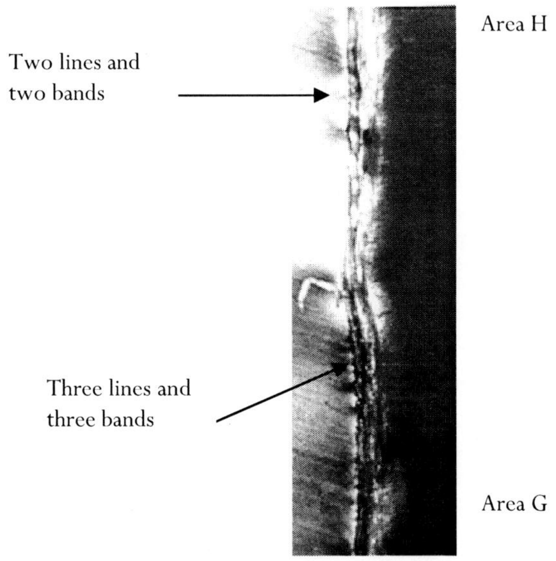

Specimen 5: 5 years 1 month, Unknown sex, Died June / July

The number of bands and lines varied between two and five depending on the location being examined. At location B there are two very broad white bands, with a broad black line in between, and a thin black line on the outer edge. At location Y the inner cementum appears to be acellular, and has five lines and five bands: on top of this is lacunae cellular cementum. The neo-natal line is very clear. The cementum on the outer edge is variable in colour: for much of the root it could be interpreted either as the beginning of a dark line or as the end of a light band, suggesting a late summer or early winter death.

Summary

It is difficult to decide what interpretation would be put on the age of this section if it were unknown. However, even if the age cannot be clearly identified, a late summer or early winter death would be very strongly suggested.

Specimen 6: 6 years 2 months, Male, Died July / August.

At location A there was one band only, while in location D there were five bands and five lines, and in locations Y and Z there were four light and four dark layers, with a light outer layer. A light outer layer was also identified at locations D and F, but the outer layer was dark at H and Y. Figure 16 is of location G, and shows a maximum of three bands and three lines.

Figure 16

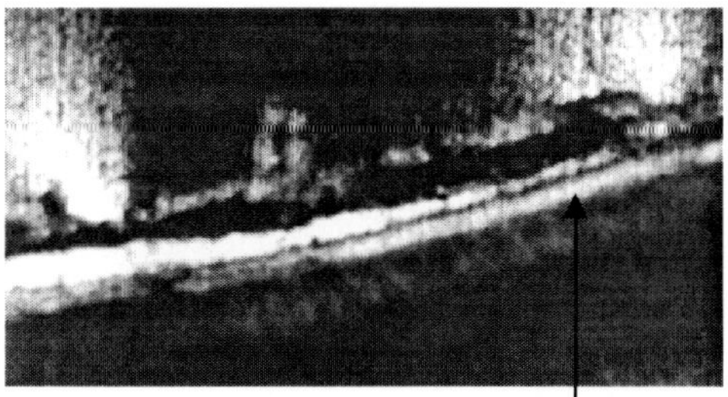

Location G showing two very clear bands and lines and a less clear band on the outer edge.

Summary

It is quite clear that no consistent age or seasonality can be assigned to this section, and that the ageing would be inaccurate whatever location was examined.

Specimen 7: 6 years 11 months, Female, Died April / May

The number of bands and lines which can be observed in different locations varies between none and six: the locations which give the closest estimate to the actual age of the tooth are B, F, and H. The outer layer is dark, suggesting a winter death: however, it varies in thickness around the root, which could suggest anything from a late summer to a late winter death. Clearly this is not sufficiently accurate for a meaningful interpretation of the season of occupation of a site. The measurement analysis undertaken by Burke (1995) would not address this problem, since the thickness varies according to the location being studied.

Specimen 8: 7 years 6 months, Unknown sex, Died November / December

This tooth could be aged accurately at location H, which exhibited 7 bands and 8 lines. However, in all of the other locations the cementum was either damaged during the animal's life, or did not show consistent layering, the number of bands and lines ranging between none and five. In the areas of damage it was common to find a single band of cellular cementum, suggesting rapid repair. The outer edge was dark in all locations except G, suggesting a winter death. Given the consistency over most of the tooth, this section would probably give rise to an accurate seasonality assessment.

The outer layer at location Y was unnaturally thick, and was also unusual in that it contained very few lacunae.

Specimen 9: 8 years 4 months, Male, Died September / October

As with most of the sections, the number of bands and lines varied between locations from none to nine. It was observed that between locations G and H there were pockets of resorbed cementum, and that cellular cementum was dominant. This suggests that the cementum in this area was under pressure, perhaps as a result of the tooth moving forward in the jaw. Between four and five bands were observed in the pad area (location Y). Figure 18 shows location B, where there seem to be five lines and six bands: a similar count is made at location F (Figure 20), and just below location E (Figure 19). At location E itself, cellular cementum can be seen overlaying the acellular cementum, although there are again five lines and six bands in the acellular cementum (Figure 17).

Summary

Given the consistency between locations B, E, and F, a confident but incorrect age assessment would probably be made for this animal.

Specimen 10: 9 years 3 months, Male, Died August / September

The number of bands and lines again varied between none and seven. Seven bands and lines could be seen at each of locations B, C, and F: since seven is the maximum number anywhere on the section, this would give rise to a very confident, but quite inaccurate, age assessment. This section was particularly interesting at location A, where there were clear double increments with two dark lines together. Resorption indicated cementum damage at location C. A light outer layer of consistent width strongly that the season of death was the end of summer. Location Y had six layers in the lacunae with a light outer edge. Figure 22 shows location H, which is commonly regarded as one of the clearest regions for incremental analysis: in this case, the cementum is mainly cellular with pockets of resorption. The same location is shown at greater magnification in Figure 21.

Summary

This section gives a clear example of the problems of cementum incremental analysis. A trained observer would confidently predict that this animal was seven years old and died in late summer.

Figure 17

Cellular cementum

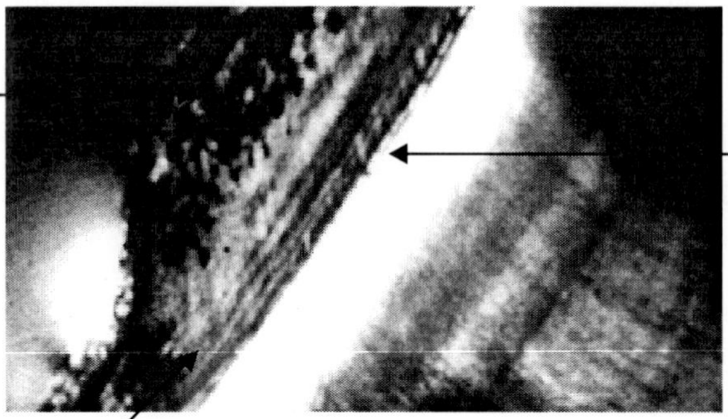

Area E where cellular cementum is overlaying acellular cementum. This is common in the area around the pad, and emphasizes the need for examiners to have an understanding of the different types of cementum for accurate analysis.

Acellular cementum

Figure 18

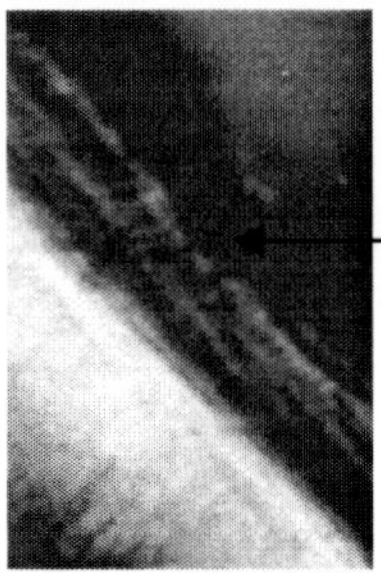

Location B showing five lines and six bands. If the bands and lines were miss counted, there are still not enough to reach the actual age of this animal. The outer edge varies even in this small area, and could not be used to interpret seasonality.

Figure 19

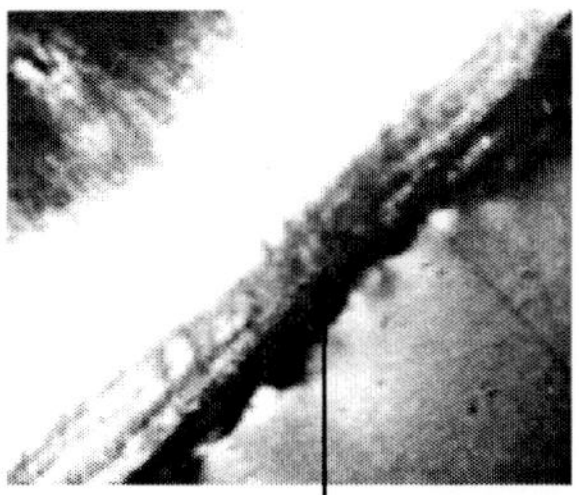

Cementum resorption, cellular cementum and lacunae present.

Figure 20

In location F there are clear bands and lines that appear grooved. There is a maximum of five bands and lines, which would again give an underestimate of age.

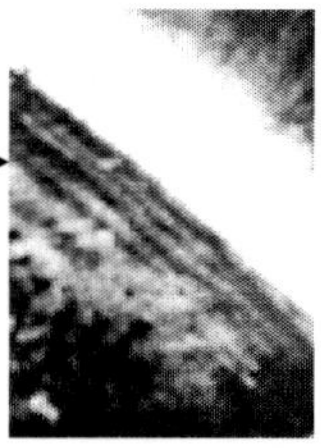

Figure 21

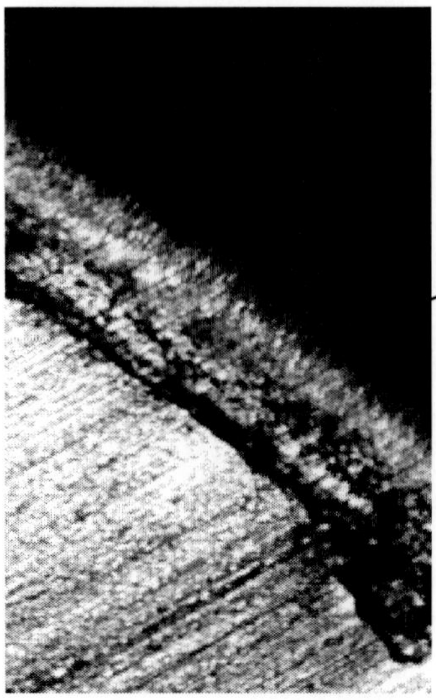

Location H
X100

Figure 22

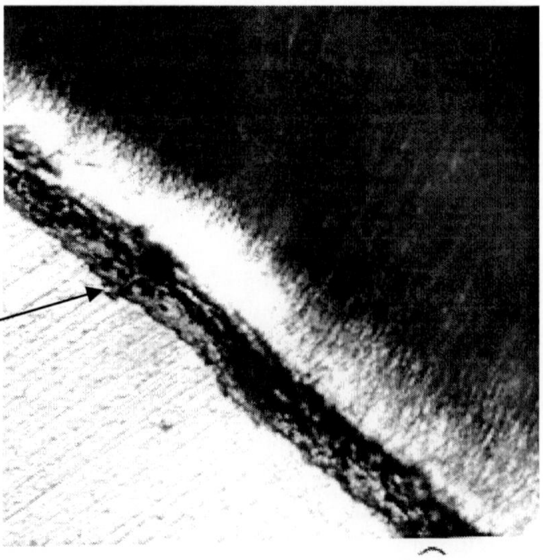

Location H
X40

Figure 23. Edge damaged at location F

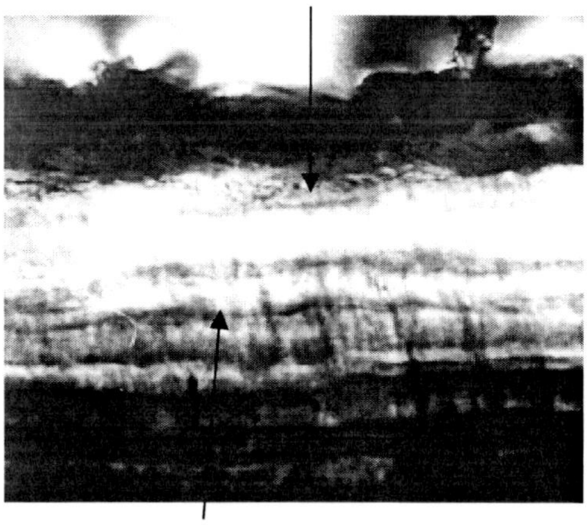

Higher magnification shows the pits and grooves in cementum, this magnification could not be used on this tooth for ageing or seasonality.

Figure 24.

Band

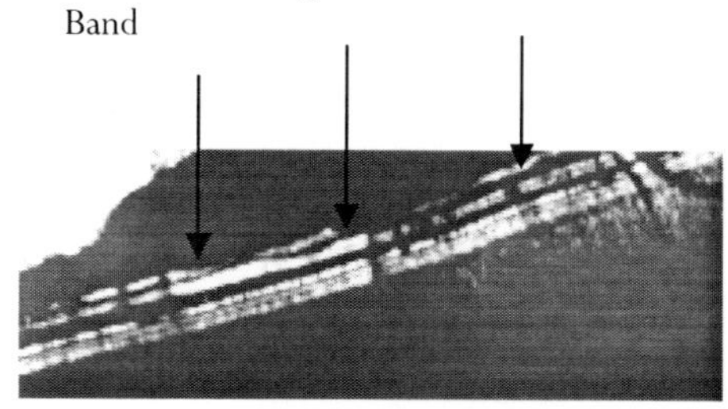

Location H

Figure 25.

Line

Band

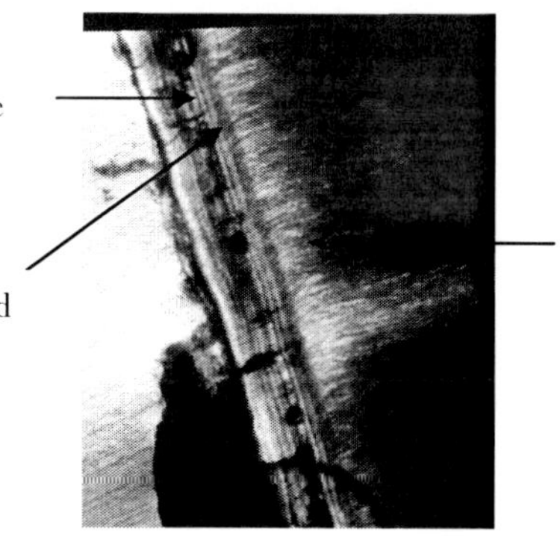

Location H

Specimen 11: 10 years 5 months, Female, Died October / November

The greatest number of bands and lines was eight, at location C. The location where the increments were clearest was H (Figure 24), although the number of bands here was not equal to the animal's age at death. Severe cementum damage was evident at location E, where the cementum had been lost to the point that the dentine was nearly completely exposed. The outer layer was light at locations F, X, Y, and Z, but distinctly dark at locations B, C, and H. In this situation one would normally interpret the seasonality as late summer or early winter, which is approximately correct. Locations X, Y, and Z show relatively clear layering, with a maximum of six pairs of lacunae bands present. Figure 25 also shows location H, where the bands and lines make a transition from being very dark to being rather lighter. Although this may be an optical effect, it seems to suggest a genuine difference in the material. The outermost cementum does not exhibit clear layering, and the very outer edge has some tissue adhering to it. This may be the result of the resin not having penetrated to the edge of the tooth due to inadequate degreasing. Figure 23 shows location F, where there are clear signs of damage to the cementum during the lifetime of the animal. This location would not be suitable for any analysis of the incremental structure.

Specimen 12: 10 years 8 months, Female, Died January / February

This tooth was damaged in many areas (locations A, E, G, and X). The greatest number of bands and lines which could be observed was at location H, where there were 4 bands and 5 lines. Seasonality was equally difficult to interpret, with the outer edge being light at locations B, C, and Y, and dark at location H. The clearest incremental structure was at location H.

Specimen 13: 13 years 8 months, Female, Died January / February

Once again, the number of bands and lines that could be distinguished varied around the tooth from none to nine. Location B was the clearest, and showed the greatest number of layers, whereas locations C and F were unreadable. At these magnifications, no layering at all could be discerned on the pad or apical cementum. The outer edge also varied around the tooth, being very dark in some locations (A, B, E, F, H, and X) and the end of a broad light band in others (C and G). Figure 26 shows a location between H and G: here there were clear layers, with six bands and lines in total. The neo-natal line is well defined. However the total number of bands and lines in the acellular cementum do not come anywhere near the real age of the animal, and any interpretation of this section would lead to a serious underestimation of the actual age. Cellular cementum overlays the acellular cementum as the pad area of the tooth is approached.

Summary

Any attempt to determine the age of this animal would be a substantial underestimate. It would be hard to make any sensible assessment of seasonality based on the section as a whole.

Specimen 14: 16 years 4 months, Female, Died September / October

This section showed clear signs of the extreme age of the animal. It was very worn, the roots were short and thick,

Figure 26. Location G to H

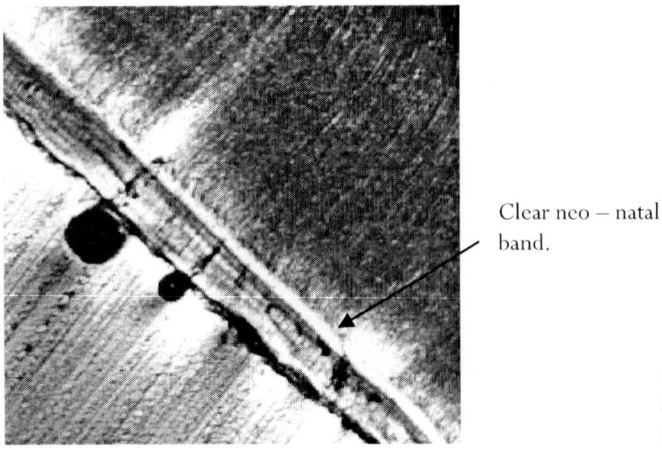

Figure 27. Location D

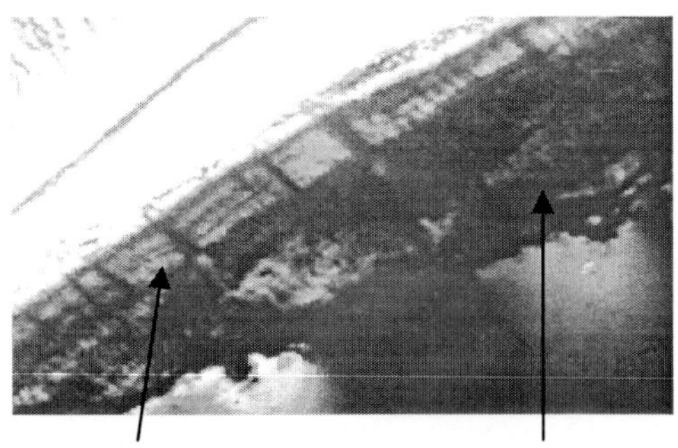

and there were resorption pockets and much cellular cementum between locations A and B, as well as a bulb/ridge of cellular cementum to compensate for dentine damage. At location A there were 5 very clear bands and 5 lines, which disappear before location B. The greatest number of bands and lines were found at location C, where there were eleven and twelve respectively. The cementum at this location was unusual, appearing as grooves and ridges. Seasonality is again difficult to interpret, with a dark layer on the edge and locations D and E, and a wide light bands at locations A, B, C, and F. Location G is shown on Figure 28 and it is clear that at this location alone there are variations in the number of bands and lines that can be counted. There is also a distinct area of resorption.

Figure 28.

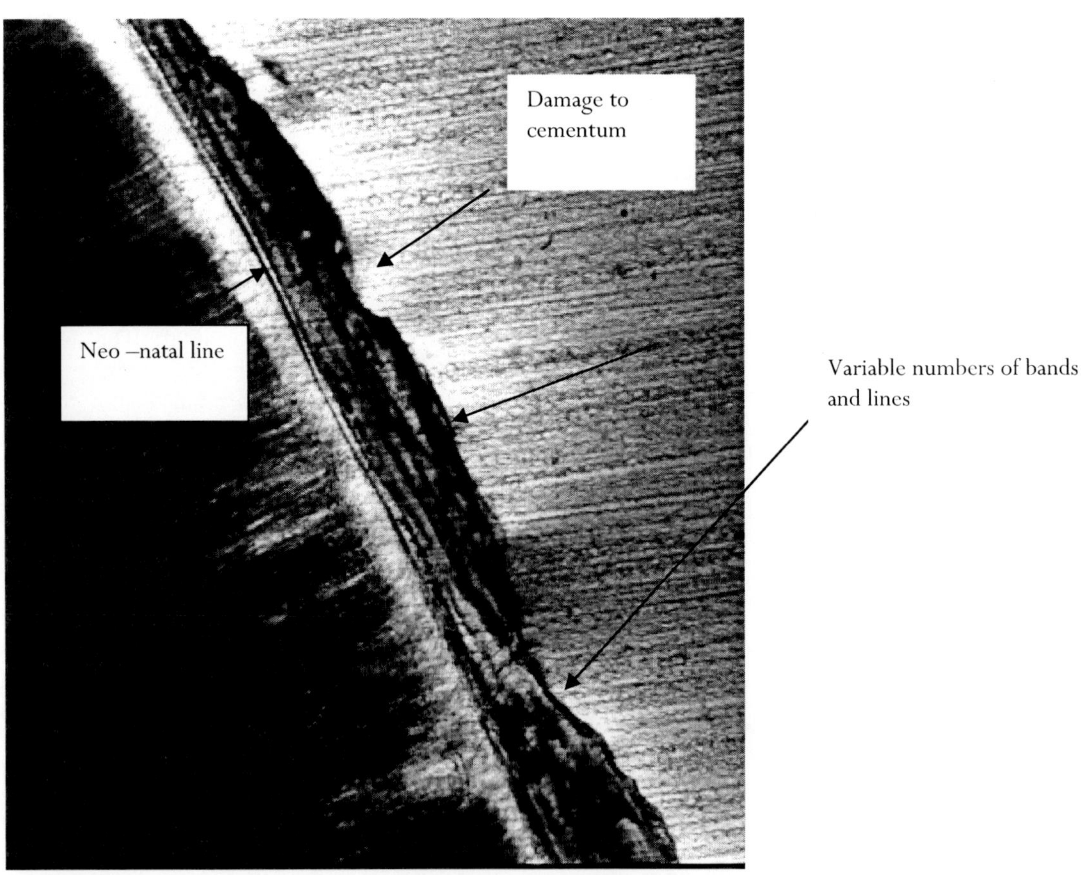

Figure 29. Dentine thickening and cementum thinning as a result.

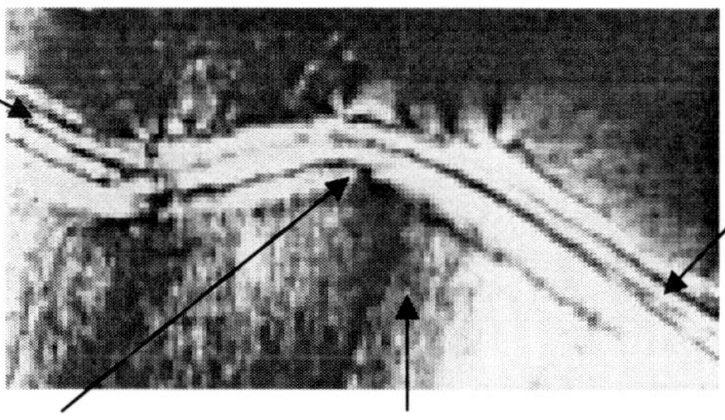

Summary

It is unlikely that any microscopical technique would reveal enough layers to make an accurate assessment of the age of this animal, or would enable a sensible estimate of seasonality.

Conclusions

Animals are individuals, and it is unsurprising that they should show substantial differences in tooth structure. Figure 29 shows a section in which the root is not straight in the area close to the crown. It can clearly be seen that there is a transition from three lines and bands to only two as the dentine becomes thicker. This supports the theory that cementum fills the gap between the dentine and the bone: where the gap is smaller, the thickness of the cementum is reduced.

In the known aged sample analysed above, there are significant variations in the distribution of cellular and acellular cementum and in the thickness of the cementum, both around a given tooth and between teeth. Adding to these differences the subjectivity of incremental analysis, I would claim that it is very unlikely that it is possible to assess seasonality, or even age, with any degree of accuracy using this technique alone.

Examination of standard ground thick sections of a modern control sample of Red deer

Thick sections are examined using reflected light microscopy. At times, the layering of the increments viewed in thick sections can be so clear that they can be examined quite satisfactorily using the naked eye. In any case, only low levels of magnification are required. The layers can be seen more clearly if they are either polished or wet (Klevezal 1996). Some researchers have used acid to etch the surface of thick sections: this makes the layers clearer (Perrin and Myrick 1980, after Klevezal 1996). For the purposes of this study etching was not attempted. For thick section examination, the pad area (i.e. the area between the roots) and the apices of the roots are the areas most commonly studied (Mitchell 1967, Koike and Ohtaishi 1985). As described in Chapter 1, the cementum found in these areas is cellular, which is produced differently to the acellular cementum which is found on the outer edges of the root. Wildlife biologists (e.g.Mitchell 1967, Lowe 1967) found this to be an accurate technique for estimating age. Mitchell (1963), (1967), claims that using facial sections, the white appearance of the cementum layers under reflected light is due to refraction from the cell cavities. The alternating broad white and narrower translucent layers are observed because the white layers are rich in cells (or cell cavities), and hence reflect more light than the translucent (cell deficient) layers. It follows that with facial sections, correct orientation of the specimen in relation to the light is important.

It is my belief that although broad estimates of age may perhaps be obtained using this method, it is not possible to assign seasonality using thick sections. The thickness of the layers in the pad and apical cementum varies to such a degree, depending on age, stress on the teeth, and nutrition, that it is impossible to estimate seasonality using cellular cementum. Also, the teeth move not only through the jaw to bring them into wear, but also forward in the jaw socket as the teeth move upwards. This is in response to the grinding of food and the need for more room to be made as the thicker area of the tooth reaches the jaw line. The cementum therefore has to be resorbed to allow for this movement, and hence it is not possible to say whether the cementum being examined is in its entirety. This movement forwards and upwards can be seen quite clearly in Figure 30 and is discussed at length at the end of this chapter.

Mitchell (1963) states that, although the rate of eruption of each tooth never completely compensates for the rate of wear of the crown, the rate of growth of cementum is clearly related to the rate of wear. For example, molariform teeth have thicker depositions of cementum than incisors or canines, and teeth showing abnormal wear have correspondingly thicker deposits.

Thick section examination was undertaken on all sections prior to the production of a thin section, and the results of the two methods were compared (see the table after the analysis of the specimens).

The thick sections described here were studied using a Leica microscope with magnification of 6.3 X and 16 X. The photographs were taken using a Leitz Wild camera attached to the microscope.

Figure 30. M1 in the bone showing differences in cementum deposition

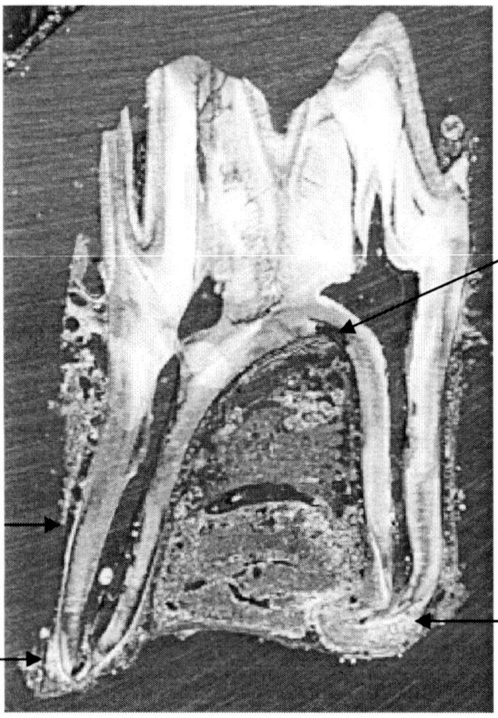

In most cases the cellular cementum is fairly regular in formation. The cementocytes within the cementum can however, be highly irregular. As with the thin sections, a great deal of subjectivity is involved in the examination, and this should be borne in mind when considering the analysis presented below.

Specimen 1: 1 year 7 months, Male, Died December / January

Figure 31 shows the pad and one of the apices. Clearly not much cementum can be expected on an animal so young, and the most accurate method of ageing would be by eruption and wear. In fact, there is no evidence of any cementum layering in this area. An interesting feature, from the point of view of incremental analysis, is that this animal, despite being so young, exhibits uneven levels of cementum distribution in the pad area. Around the rest of the root the cementum appears to be continuous.

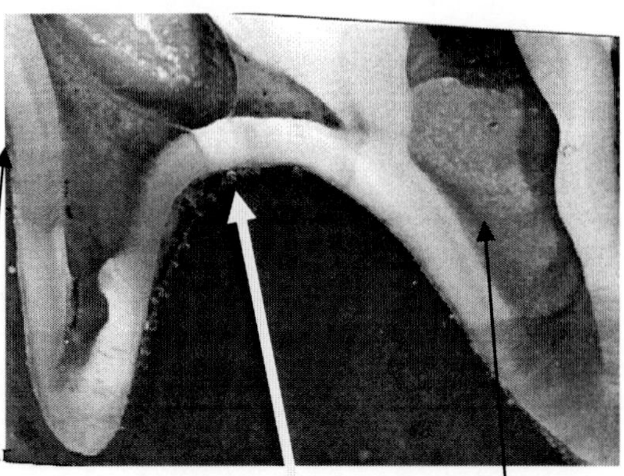

Figure 31. Uneven cellular cement in the pad area

Specimen 2: 2 years 8 months, Male, Died January / February

In this section, apical cementum had begun to form on one root (Figure 32). The pad cementum is uneven in distribution in this area, but could be interpreted with reasonable accuracy for ageing.

Specimen 3: 3 years 7 months, Female, Died December / January

Figure 33 shows the pad of this tooth. This might be interpreted as exhibiting two thick bands and two lines, although on closer examination up to four bands might be observed. It is clear, however, that no reasonable assessment of seasonality could be made in this area.

Figure 32. Cementum of Red deer aged 2 years 8 months

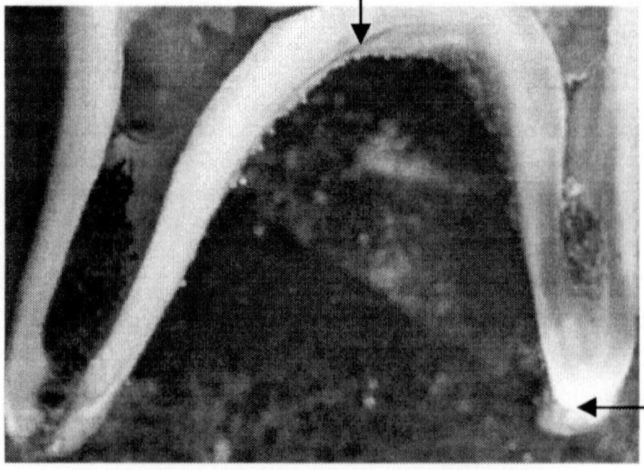

Figure 33. Pad cementum of M1 of Red deer aged 3 years 7 months

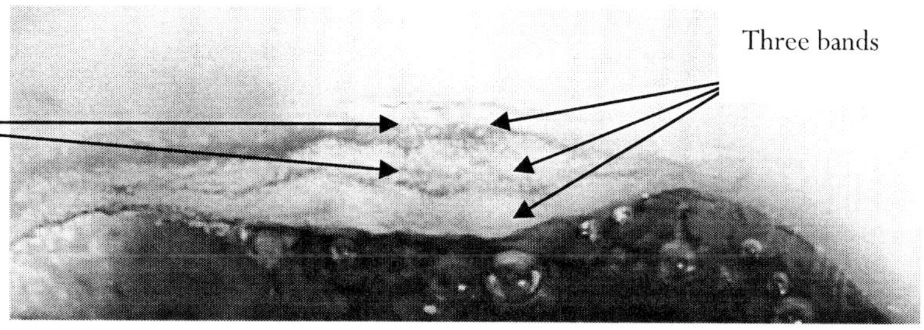

Fig 34. Pad cementum of a M1 of a Red deer aged 4 years 5 months

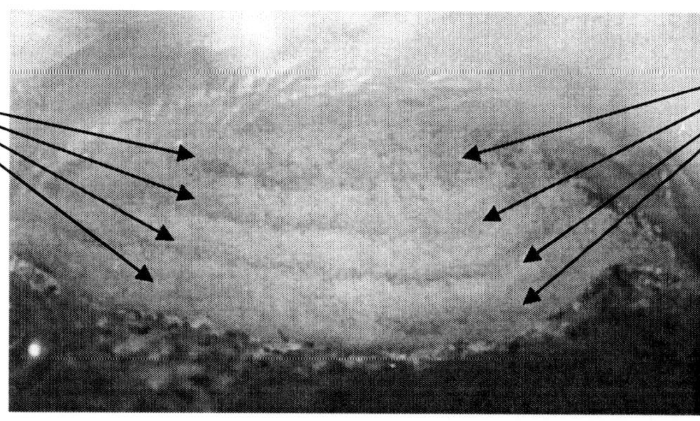

Figure 35. Close up of pad cementum of M1 of Red deer aged 5 years 1 month

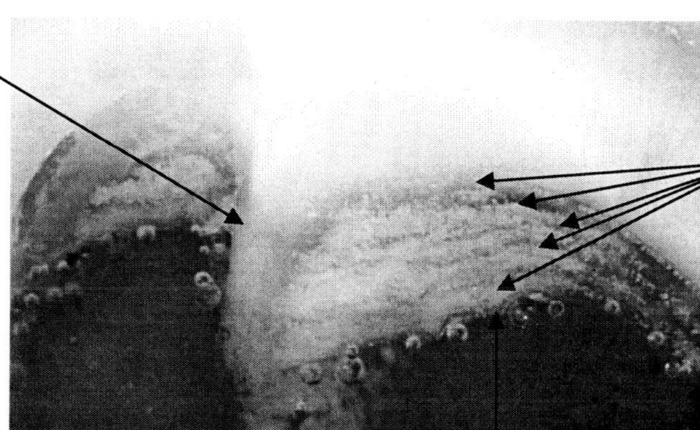

Figure 36. Pad cementum of M1 of a Red deer aged 6 years 2 months

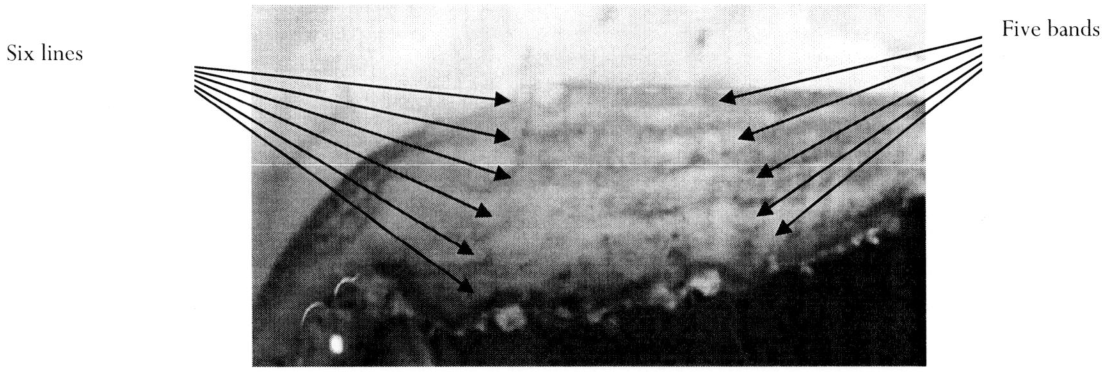

Specimen 4: 4 years 5 months, Female, Died October / November

Four lines and five bands can be clearly discerned on this specimen, leading to an accurate assessment of age.

Specimen 5: 5 years 1 month, Unknown sex, Died June / July

As has already been mentioned, highly individual features can be observed in certain animals: Figure 35 shows a close up of the pad of this animal which exhibits an extra region of dentine: this is a relatively uncommon feature. In the larger region of cementum there are five clear bands and lines, and it might even be suggested that the outer layer is a line, indicating a winter death. This interpretation would be inaccurate, given that the animal died in summer.

Specimen 6: 6 years 2 months, Male, Died July / August

Figure 36 shows this thick section. The outer layer would be difficult to assess for seasonality, but there appear to be five bands and six lines, so that a relatively accurate assessment of age could be made from this section.

Specimen 8: 7 years 6 months, Unknown sex, Died November / December

Figure 37 shows no consistent layers. The cellular cementum is full of cementocytes, and is not useful for age or seasonality assessment. The very edge of the pad appears to have undergone some resorption.

Figure 37. M1 pad cementum of Red deer aged 7 years 6 months

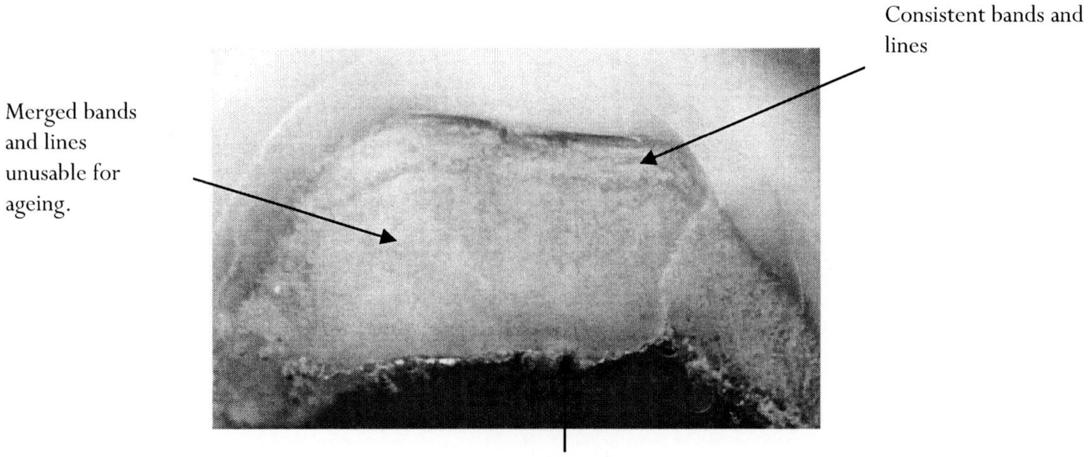

Figure 38. Close up of pad cementum of M1 of a Red deer aged 8 years 4 months

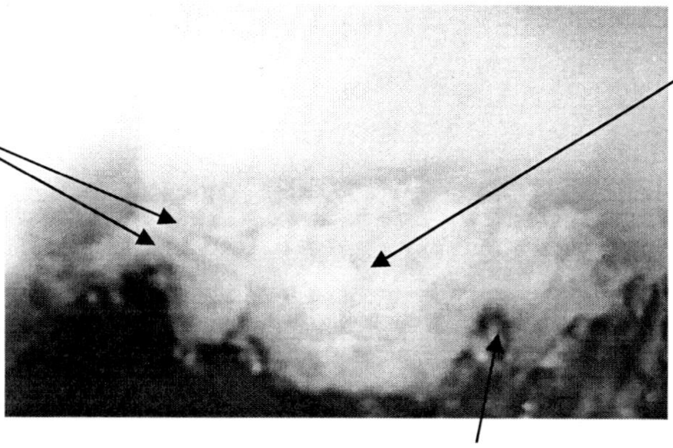

Specimen 9: 8 years 4 months, Male, Died September / October

This section (Figure 38) exhibits very uneven cellular cementum, with clear areas of localised resorption. Five bands and lines can be identified, giving rise to a substantial underestimate of age. Animals which are adult but not very old (i.e. under 10 years) are the hardest for wildlife biologists to age accurately. Unfortunately this section would not prove very helpful in ageing this animal.

Specimen 10: 9 years 3 months, Male, Died August / September

This section is shown in Figure 39. It is interesting to note that, although the cementum pad is very thick, there is little acellular cementum on the lower half of the root. Notice the unevenness of the bottom edge of the pad, which would give rise to an inaccurate seasonality assessment. There are, however, nine bands and nine lines which can be distinguished reasonably clearly, so ageing would be accurate (allowing for interpretative differences between observers).

Figure 39. Root and pad cementum of a M1 of a Red deer aged 9 years 3 months

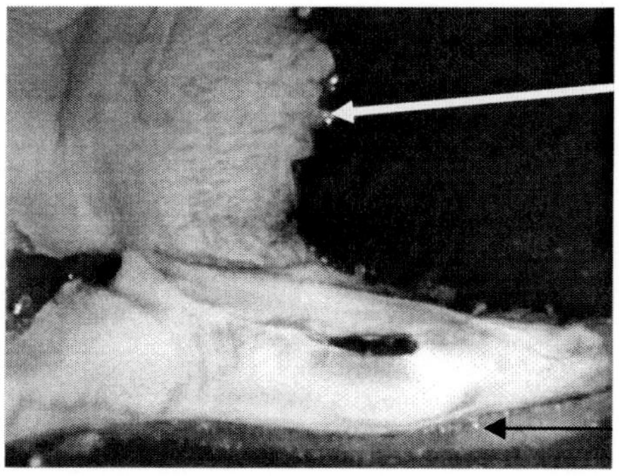

Specimen 11: 10 years 5 months, Female, Died October / November

Ten bands and ten lines, all reasonably regular and clear, can be identified on this pad (Figure 40). An accurate age assessment could therefore be made.

Specimen 13: 13 years 8 months, Female, Died January / February

At the edge of the pad there are twelve lines and twelve bands (Figure 41). However, more can be discerned in the middle of the pad, and the number is not always consistent – the age assessment is therefore open to interpretation. An experienced observer would probably be able to make a reasonable assessment of age from this section. As with all the thick sections, seasonality assessment would be very difficult.

Specimen 14: 16 years 4 months, Female, Died September / October

Figure 42 shows the roots and pad of this particularly old animal. It is clear that the apical cementum would not be useable to make an age assessment, and that the acellular cementum on the inner edges of the root has all but disappeared. The pad cementum exhibits up to ten bands and lines at this magnification, which would clearly give rise to a substantial underestimate of the true age of the animal. Photograph 43 shows a close up of the pad area, in which up to twelve bands and lines can be discerned. It is interesting to note that towards the end of the life of this animal, the bottom of the pad area is transparent, indicating that the cementum is less dense.

Figure 40. Close up of pad cementum of a Red deer M1 aged 10 years and 5 months

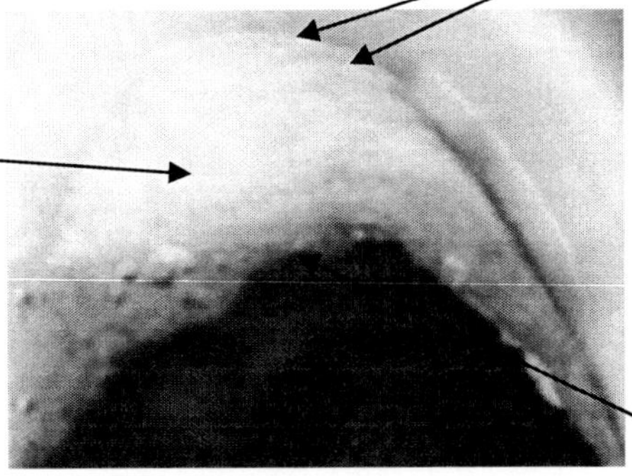

Figure 41. Close up of pad cementum of M1 of a Red deer aged 13 years and 8 months

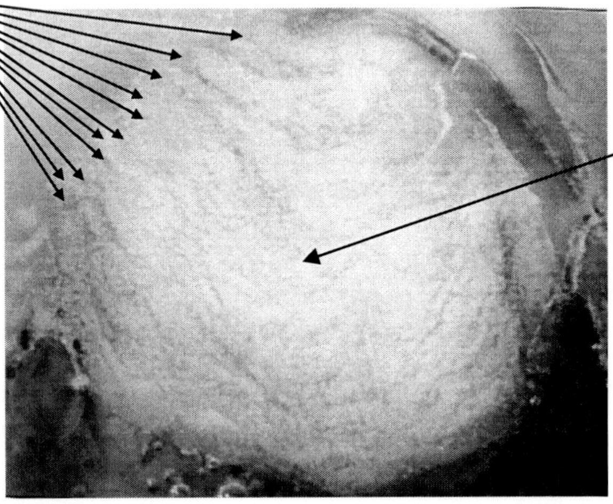

Figure 42. Pad cementum of Red deer aged 16 years 4 months

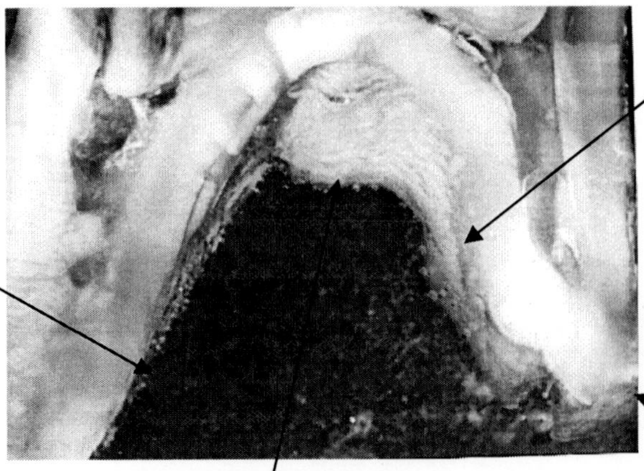

Figure 43. Close up of pad of Red deer aged 16 years 4 months

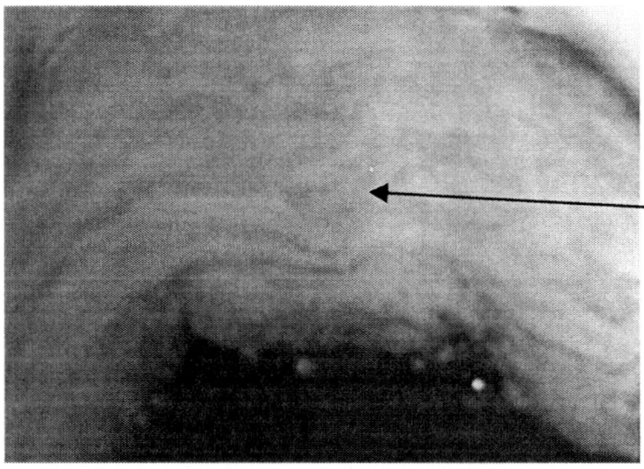

Known age (M1)	Age in years from thin section	Age in years from thick section
1 year 7 months	Between 2 and 3	Unreadable
2 years 8 months	Between 4 and 5	Between 2 and 3
3 years 7 months	Between 5 and 6	Between 2 and 4
5 years 1 month	Between 2 and 5	5
6 years 2 months	Between 3 and 5	6
7 years 6 months	Between 5 and 8	Unreadable
8 years 4 months	Up to 9	5
9 years 3 months	Up to 7	9
10 years 5 months	Up to 8	10
13 years 8 months	Up to 9	13
16 years 4 months	Up to 12	Up to 12

Table 5: Analysis of the modern control sample.

Conclusions

The table above summarises the age assessments which would be made for each section on the basis of analysis of the thin and thick sections.

It is apparent from this table that age assessments from thick sections are in fact considerably more accurate than those from thin sections. Even here, however, the errors are sufficiently great that it would be difficult to have confidence that an animal of unknown age had been aged more than approximately (to within three years, say). No accurate seasonality determination appears to be possible from either thin or thick sections: the very few cases in which an accurate seasonality assessment has been made can easily be attributed to chance.

5. RELIABILITY OF CEMENTUM INCREMENTAL ANALYSIS

A statistical study was carried out, in an attempt to determine both the intraexaminer and interexaminer reliability of cementum incremental analysis: that is, how reliably a trained examiner can replicate his measurements on a given section, and how reliably two different examiners can arrive at the same measurements when studying the same section. The theoretical basis of this study, which uses the *intraclass correlation coefficient of reliability (ICC)* is described in detail in Chapter 7, where it is applied to a scoring scheme for age determination; a step by step tutorial guide to carrying out the technique can also be found in Appendix 5. It should be stressed that the issue of reliability is quite separate from that of accuracy: no attempt is made here to consider how accurate an examiner's age estimations are, simply how reliably he can replicate them. The reason for deferring a full discussion of the method until Chapter 7 is that a far more detailed reliability analysis can be applied to the scoring scheme, simply because both intraexaminer and interexaminer reliability of the scoring scheme are excellent, whereas the intraexaminer reliability of cementum incremental analysis is so poor that any consideration of interexaminer reliability, or indeed of accuracy, becomes meaningless. In other words, a single examiner, studying the same thin section on different occasions, arrives at such widely varying interpretations of what he sees that it is not sensible to ask how well these measurements correlate with the true age of the jaw, or with those of a second, and equally unreliable, examiner. This reliability study therefore provides one of the principal objections to the technique of cementum incremental analysis, providing a statistical demonstration that the various difficulties involved with the technique, which have already been described in detail, are so great as to make it unworkable.

Method and Results

The sample used consisted of thin sections of twelve M1s which have already been discussed in this chapter. Each of the sections was examined carefully under polarised transmitted light on two separate occasions, separated by at least six months, by each of two trained examiners, the author (examiner 1) and Dr. W. A. B. Brown, a dental anatomist (examiner 2). Each section was studied in eleven different locations, as indicated in Figure 14, and in each such location where the tooth was not damaged and the section was readable, the number of bands and lines was recorded. From these readings, each examiner also made a best possible estimate of the age in years of the animal under study. As has been explained, this is not in general an easy task, since the incremental structure varies so widely at different locations on the tooth. Where possible, the estimate was usually based upon the number of bands and lines at locations A and H.

Intraexaminer reliability studies were then carried out for each of the two examiners, on each of the following data: reliability of age estimation; reliability of counting bands; and reliability of counting lines. The intraexaminer reliability in all of these categories was found to be so poor that it was decided that there was no point in proceeding to an analysis of interexaminer reliability – if an examiner cannot reliably replicate his own measurements, then they cannot be sensibly compared with those of another examiner.

The following results were obtained upon carrying out a reliability analysis as described in Chapter 7 and Appendix 5:

Category	Examiner 1	Examiner 2
Age Estimate	42.2%	22.1%
Band Counting	27.4%	51.5%
Line Counting	30.2%	51.5%

Table 6: Reliability of cementum incremental analysis

All of these reliabilities are poor, especially when compared with those of the scoring scheme. The most probable explanation of the observation that examiner 2, while having a higher reliability than examiner 1 in counting bands and lines, had a substantially lower reliability in age estimation, is that he was much more likely than examiner 1 to mark a location as unreadable when there was any doubt as to the interpretation. This tends to increase the reliability of counting increments, but clearly does not contribute to a more reliable age estimation.

6. EXAMINATION OF CEMENTUM WHILE STILL IN THE JAW USING X RAY ANALYSIS

In order to attempt to examine the function of cementum it decided that the cementum should be examined while still in the jaw. By doing this it was hoped that it would be possible to identify whether a) the cementum reacts to wear on the tooth (so the teeth are moving through the socket by a biological mechanism, and the cementum is laid down to prevent a space forming between the bone and the tooth root); or b) that the teeth are forced into wear by the deposition of cementum. This issue has already been discussed in Chapter 1. Essentially there is no agreement about the role of additive cementum (Jones 1997). Teeth erupt as soon as the root commences to be formed, long before the apex of the tooth is complete: that is, they erupt without any apical cementum being present. It would therefore seem sensible to suggest that cementum is reacting to tooth wear by filling the gap left as the tooth root moves out of the socket: without this cementum deposition, the tooth would become unstable as it moved into wear and could not function properly.

Teeth erupt at the same time that the jaw is growing. A bony socket forms around the tooth, which moves towards functional occlusion with the teeth of the opposing jaw and away from the lower border of the mandible: at this stage the socket bone remodels to form a hard casting of bone around the tooth. The periodontal ligament (discussed in Chapter 1) acts as a cushion and securing mechanism for the tooth.

Materials and methods

A collection of 24 known aged lower jaws from Scotland, covering all ages from 5 months old to 16 years, were X-rayed before any teeth were removed for incremental analysis. I am very grateful to Patsy Whelehan of the Department of Veterinary Medicine Cambridge, who took the X rays.

Figure 44: X Ray analysis of cementum of the teeth while still in the jaw

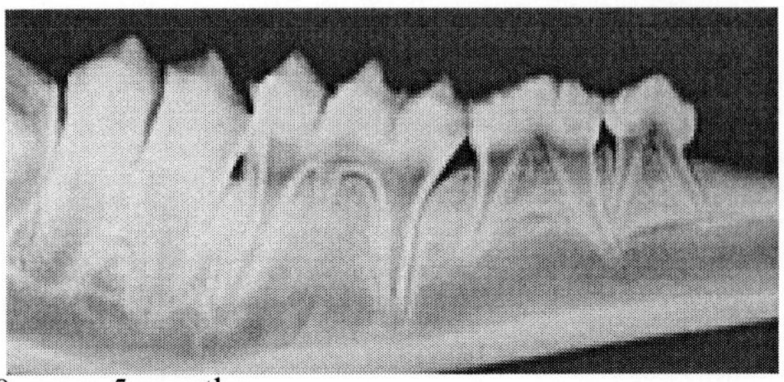

0 years 5 months

0 years 5 months

The deciduous M1 has just erupted. The roots are long, reaching the bottom of the bone. All of the apices of the tooth roots are open

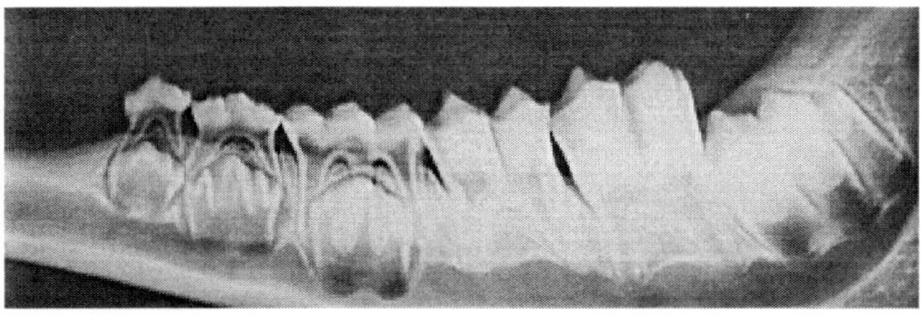

1 year 7 months

1 year and 7 months
The third molar has yet to erupt. The second molar has wide open roots.
The permanent premolars can be seen beneath the deciduous premolars. Bone surrounds the teeth and no cementum is present.

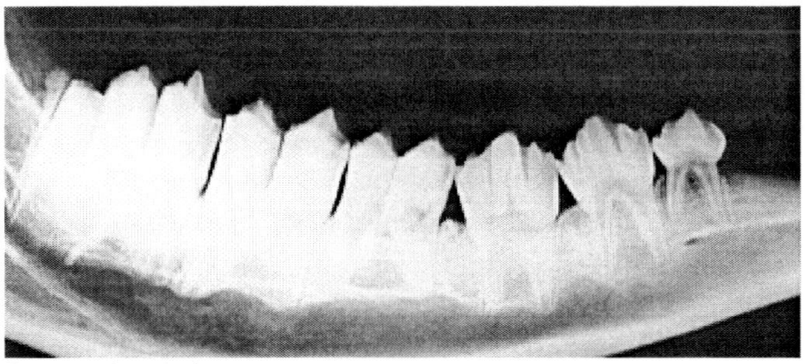

2 years 6 months

2 years 6 months
The third molar has nearly fully erupted. The hypoconulid is still only just cutting through the bone. The permanent premolars have fully erupted. The bone still encases the teeth; very little cementum is present.

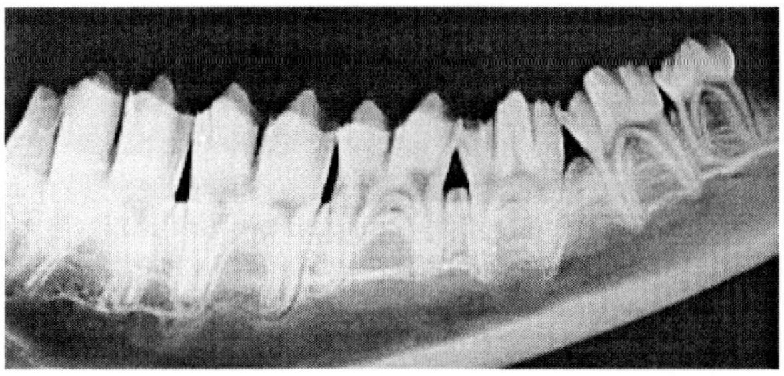

3 years 7 months

3 years 7 months
The hypoconulid of the third molar is now fully erupted and will be in wear. The pulp cavity of the first and second molar is beginning to fill with dentine.
The third molar still shows open roots. The bone is still encasing the roots, though cementum can now be seen. The M1 shows quite a thick cementum pad as the tooth has moved into wear

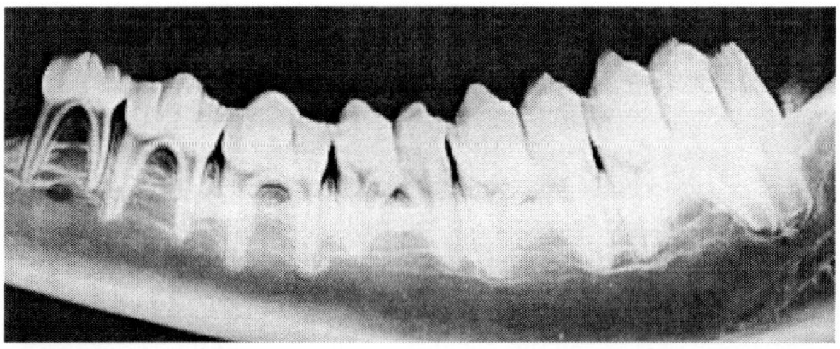

4 years 5 months

4 years 5 months
The first molar is moving up through the bone to keep the tooth in wear. Cementum is forming quite thickly on the apices. The hypoconulid root and one root of the third molar still have to close completely.

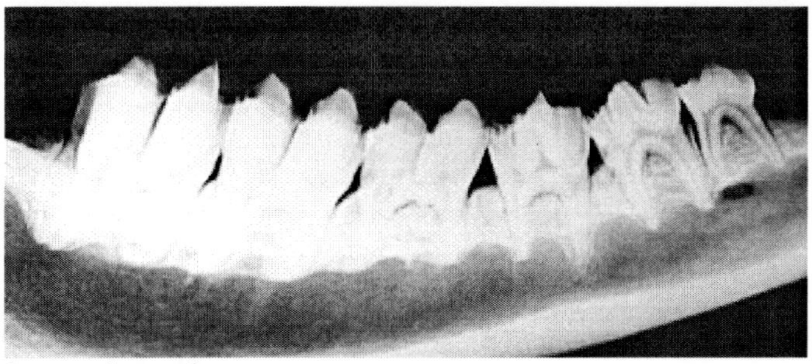

5 years 1 months

5 years 1 month
All teeth are starting to move mesially in compensation for wear. Cementum can be seen on the apices of the first and second molars, keeping the teeth in wear, filling the gap between the bone and the tooth. The bone has clearly stopped modelling around the roots.

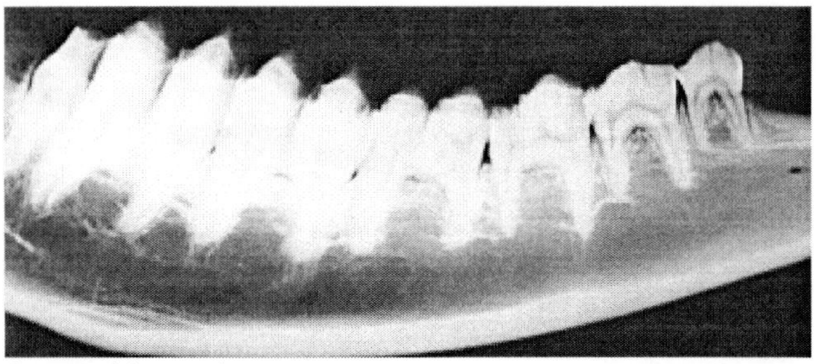

6 years 11 months

6 years 11 months

Thick cementum can be identified on the roots. The pad cementum is thick and even. The apices of the M1 suggest that this tooth is moving mesially. Note the trailing cementum filling the gap in the bone left as the tooth has migrated. There is very little evidence of the pulp cavity on M1 or M2, suggesting that it is full of dentine.

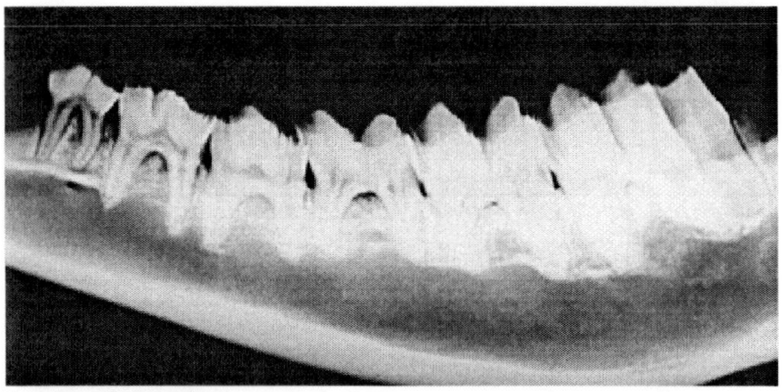

7 years 4 months

7 years 4 months

The molars have moved quite a distance through the bone. The pulp cavity is almost entirely disappeared. The M3 now demonstrates thick pad cementum.

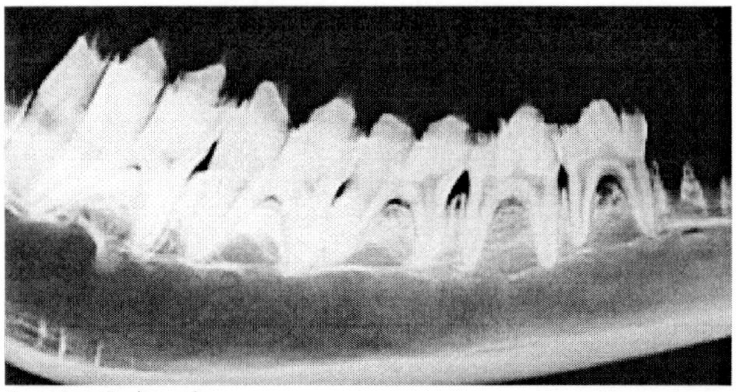

8 years 3 months

8 years 3 months

The M1 and M2 have migrated mesially with cementum being added to the apices to fill the gaps remaining between the teeth and the bones. The pad cementum distribution between the M1 and the M2 differs quite considerably as they move at different rates. This is clearly important when examining isolated teeth.

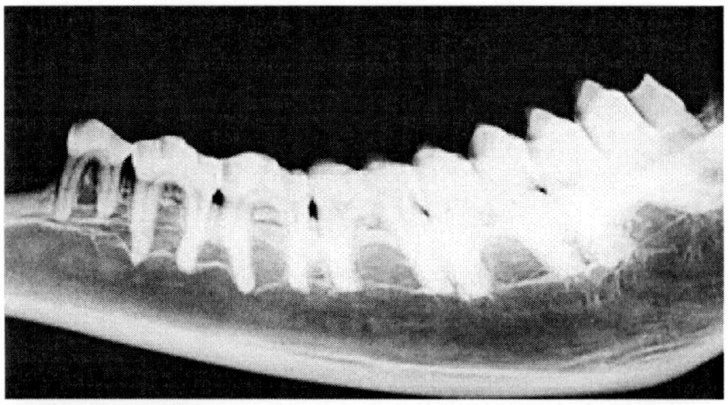

9 years 5 months

9 years 5 months

The crown of the M1 is very flat, so this tooth is well worn. This is reflected by the amount of cementum visible in the pad area and along the distal edge of the tooth.

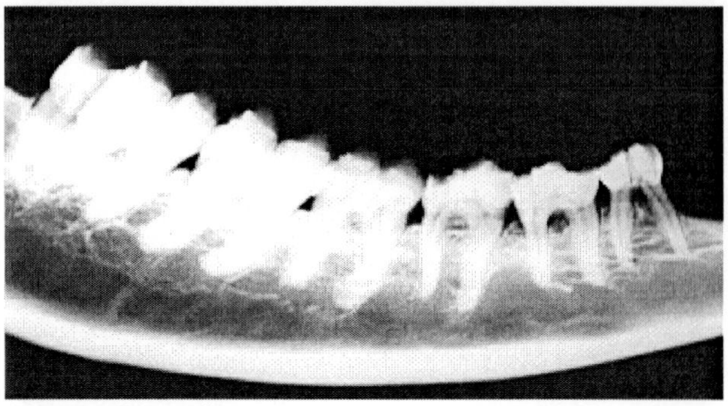

10 years 8 months

10 years 8 months

The M1 and M2 show severe movement. Notice the curling and trailing of the cementum on the apices of the roots of these teeth. Very little cementum can be identified on the mesial edge of the M1, suggesting it has been resorbed to allow for the required movement. Cementum has been deposited on the internal edge of the root on the mesial root as the tooth has moved. Cementum around this tooth is therefore very variable.

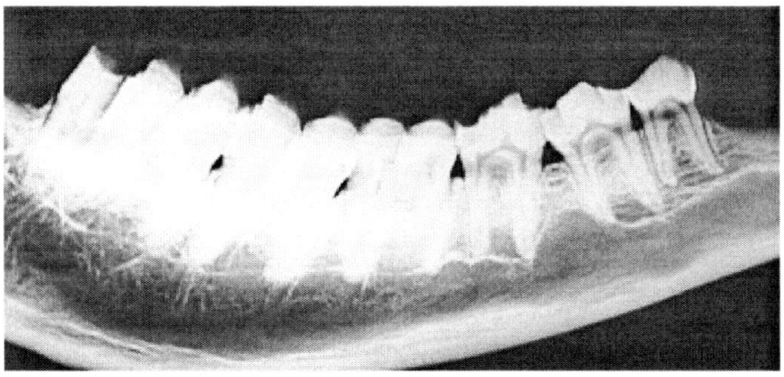

11 years 6 months

11 years 6 months
There is less trailing of the cementum on the roots of the molars of this animal. This could suggest less wear is taking place and therefore the movement is not required to the same extent.

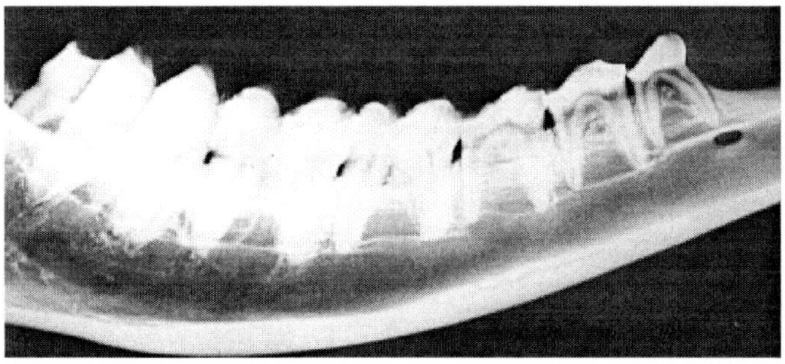

13 years 8 months

13 years 8 months
Thick cementum can be identified on all the molars. The teeth are close together and enamel has worn where the teeth meet.

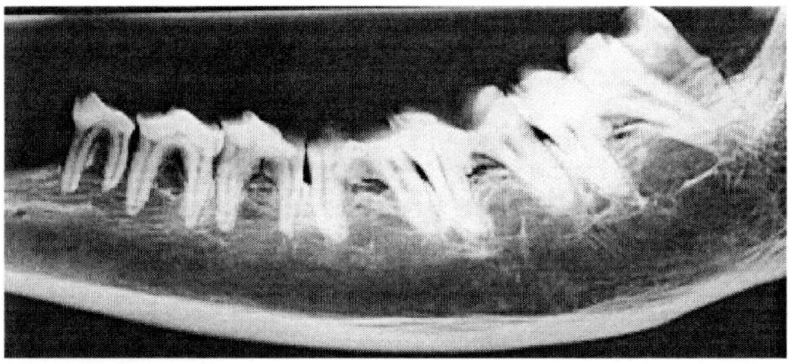

14 years 8 months

14 years 8 months
The crowns have all worn and very thick pad cementum can be seen on the M1. However, very little cementum can be identified on the mesial edge of the M1.

Discussion

Cementum appears to be a responsive element: it is laid down upon movement of the tooth through the jaw, rather than causing that movement. As mesial migration occurs, cementum is resorbed on the mesial side of the tooth, and deposited on the distal side to fill the ensuing gap. This mechanism has serious implications for accurate incremental analysis of older animals. It also seems clear that pad cementum is not evenly distributed between the first and second molars. Although this is not a problem in itself, it adds a further complication to the analysis of isolated teeth from archaeological collections, since it is very difficult to distinguish whether an isolated tooth is a first or second molar.

As has already been discussed, the distribution of cementum around the tooth root has to vary in order for the tooth to function and react to wear. It is therefore unsurprising that accurate age estimates cannot be obtained from every area of every tooth.

To confirm the way in which teeth move through the jaw and the function of cementum it was decided that the teeth should be measured. I am very grateful to Dr.W.A.B. Brown, who took measurements of all these radiographs.

The measurements were as follows:

1. The height of the mandible from the lower border of the mandibular bone (bottom of the jawbone) to the alveolar crest between the fourth premolar and the first molar. In the cases of suspected of bone loss from periodontal disease the measurement was taken to the lowest contact point between the distal surface of the premolar and the mesial surface of the molar. This measurement was to determine at what age vertical height of the mandible is achieved.
2. The height from the lowest border of the mandibular body to the lowest point on the apex of the mesial root of the first molar (the lowest point of the tooth socket). This is to determine if the distance between the lower boarder of the mandible and the lowest point of the socket increases with age.

3. The horizontal length of the three premolars and the three molars measured from the root and crown junction at the anterior edge of the mesial root of the second premolar and the root and crown junction of the most distal aspect of the third molar (mandibular

tooth row length). This is to determine if the total length shortens with age. This would be an obvious assumption given that teeth wear through contact with each other. As the wear progresses, the teeth migrate mesially to keep the teeth in contact. This contact wear is at least 2mm for the third and fourth premolar and the first and second molar and 1 mm for the second premolar and third molar. This means that the tooth row is shortened by four years. Though this may happen, the tooth root remains tight in the socket. This implies that in the process of mesial migration, the cementum of the socket is resorbed on the mesial side of the socket and added onto the distal surface, and remodelled on the lingual and buccal aspects. This would clearly affect cementum incremental analysis in terms of which area of the tooth should be looked at and the consistency of tooth around the root. This is summed up by Jones (pers. comm. 1997) who notes that there is no general agreement about the role of additive cementum in assisting eruption by simple accretion. It could be that the tooth erupts and the cementum is added on at the apices and pad to fill the space in the socket. It is probable that this accretion of cementum is to help stabilise the tooth as it erupts. Eruption is part mesial, part vertical, and part buccal. As indicated in Chapter 1 it could be that the cementum is formed to protect the dentine (Jones in Olsen ed. 1981) this accords with the evidence of the radiographs: that as the teeth are moving it is the cementum rather than the dentine which is resorbed. Thus the dentine, the core of the root, is protected from remodelling.

Conclusions

- The vertical height of the body of the mandible is achieved by three and a half years.
- The apical level of the socket after vertical height of the mandible is achieved does not change in relation to the lower border of the mandible. Therefore as the tooth continues to erupt incremental padding layers of cementum are laid down to maintain its stability within the mandible.

7. MICROSCOPY

The importance of understanding both the nature of cementum and the mechanism of section preparation before attempting any interpretation of incremental structures has already been emphasised. Equally important is a thorough understanding of. There are many variables that can affect what is seen through the microscope, especially as what is being observed is essentially light dependant. Too many interpretations have been placed on incremental bands by researchers who have no understanding or appreciation of microscopical technique, and too often the researcher is looking for the 'optimum' number of bands in given locations, when what is actually being seen is optical distortion caused either by bad section preparation or by contrast arising from improper use of the condenser or light and dark fields. This is why many researchers have emphasised the need for experience in this field before any interpretation can be undertaken with integrity. Pike-Tay (1991) notes "that it is absolutely essential that the researcher be highly experienced through practice with known age and season of death specimens. Unfamiliarity with subtleties inherent in polarised light microscopy, as well as visual distinctions between, for example, the last rest line, what was once periodontal tissue, and dirt clinging to the surrounding epoxy of a partially mineralised specimen, and viewed in "black and white" may well result in inaccurate determinations".

All of the sections that were produced for this study were looked at as bulk/thick sections under reflected light and as thin sections using polarised microscopy. Other researchers have, however, used alternative methods of microscopy for the interpretation of increments. Burke (1992) used a control sample of horse to compare polarised light microscopy with various other examination techniques, including decalcification with staining, transmitted electron microscopy, scanning electron microscopy, histochemical analysis, and microadiography. The comparison consisted of 1 tooth being subjected to microradiography, 3 to SEM, 5 to decalcification and 31(representing 16 animals) being examined under polarised transmitted light.

Polarising Microscopy

This type of microscope is distinguished by having polarising filters above and below the stage. These are arranged so that their planes of vibration are at right angles to one another (Hillson 1986). When sections are viewed under polarised light, the increments appear as alternating translucent bands and opaque bands (petrographic section). The luminance of the different bands is the result of the crystalline orientation relative to the plane of the polarised light; what is represented in the incremental pattern is differences in the physical orientation of the hydroxyaptite crystals. Thus the increment patterns seen with polarised transmitted light are the result of the physical structure of the inorganic components of the tooth cementum (Landon 1993).

Many researchers use polarised light for the examination of ground thin sections (not decalcified). Images are produced in a polarising microscope by the phenomenon of birefringence, or double refraction. (Hillson 1986). Undecalcified polarised thin sections of cement show a layer structure of different path densities, i.e. brightness (Schmidt and Keil 1972). These changes correspond to changes in the orientation of constituent collagen fibres, betraying an adjustment in the direction of growth (Burke 1992). Most minerals and many large organic structures refract a beam of light into two separate beams. Each emergent beam has a different refractive index, and is polarised. In the apatites and collagen of dental tissues, one emergent beam is polarised parallel to the optical axis of the crystal or molecule, and the other in a plane perpendicular to the axis. This arrangement is called uniaxial. The difference in refractive index between the beams is the birefringence. In apatites this ranges from

0.003 to - 0.004. Birefringence of collagen fibrils is positive, but the actual value is difficult to determine for collagen on its own. The birefringence of a mineral or organic structure also varies with orientation (Hillson 1986).

Ordinary light / Reflected light

Polished "thick sections" (see Chapter 3) can be viewed under ordinary or reflected light to reveal a pattern of alternating bright bands corresponding darker lines. Mitchell (1963, 1967) claims that using facial sections the white appearance of the cement layers under reflected light is due to refraction from the cell cavities. The alternating broad white and narrower translucent layers are seen because the white layers are rich in cells (or cell cavities), and hence reflect more light than the translucent (cell deficient) layers. Hence with facial sections, correct orientation of the specimen in relation to the light is important.

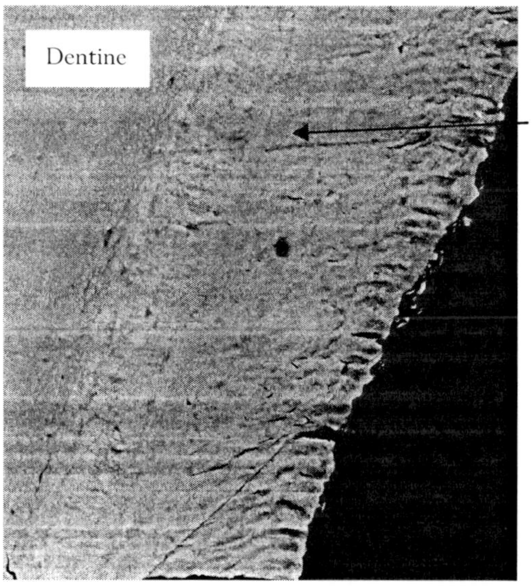

Figure 45: SEM of a Red deer first molar from Suffolk

Scanning Electron Microscopy

SEM was attempted on various teeth in order to identify different methods of examination and to understand if it was the method of sectioning, rather than the inherent difficulties of cementum incremental analysis that was at issue. Hillson (1986) also suggests that it is an accurate method of analysis. Burke (1995) used SEM analysis on a couple of her modern control samples and found that increments could be viewed using this method. It was therefore decided to test this theory on a number of sections produced for this study.

SEM was undertaken on 6 teeth that represented 5 different months of death,[2] by the Multi-Imaging Centre, Cambridge, using the Philips XL30 microscope. The samples for SEM were produced in the same way as the thick sections (see Chapter 3). They were then etched in the imaging centre to ensure the grooves and ridges could be seen. SEM was only tentatively examined, as time did not allow a more detailed examination of the value of the technique. For more information on SEM analysis of teeth see Bell, Boyde and Jones (1991), Hillson (1988) and Olsen (1988).

Figure 45 shows an SEM image of a Red deer first molar from Euston in Suffolk, which is taken from location D. The dentine and cementum can be clearly identified, and are labelled on the figure, but there is too much detail for the increments to be counted. A lower magnification might address this problem.

Computer image enhancement

This has been used as a method of examining tooth thin sections for incremental analysis by a number of researchers (for example Lieberman and Meadow 1992, Burke 1995). The technique involves taking a microscopic image, producing a digitised image of it and using an image analysis program (such as IMAGE) to view the image on a computer. A program such as IMAGE can graph the relative luminance (brightness) of pixels across the cementum increments to quantify the number of bands, and to determine whether the outermost band is opaque or translucent. Opaque bands appear as peaks and translucent bands as troughs, allowing one to calculate precisely the number and nature of increments at selected regions of the tooth root (Lieberman and Meadow 1992). Multiple transects provide rapid syntheses of information on large regions of the tooth and are particularly useful for discriminating split lines or false increments.

Computer image enhancement requires the digitisation of a microscope image. They used a Macintosh II computer using Mass Micro Colour Space II digitizer in a 640 x 480 - pixel PICT format providing a range of 256 grey levels per pixel. Once digitised, images can be filtered by a variety of functions that can increase the contrast between regions of similar pixel values. The public domain software created by Wayne Rasband of the National Institutes of Health was used to enhance some images. Computer image analysis is also useful for quantifying the results and reducing the subjectivity that has often plagued the interpretation of cementum increments.

Computer image enhancement was tested on a number of thin sections in the course of this research. I am most grateful to Neil Brodie of the McDonald Institute for Archaeological Research for his assistance with this technique.

Photographs of the thin sections were taken and scanned using Adobe Photoshop. The dimensions of the image and the number of dots per inch are recorded. These were transferred to NIH image for computer image enhancement. Several images were successfully scanned,

[2]Teeth used for SEM: 3 from Abernethy Scotland, two males and one female.

and within NIH Image it is possible to measure the width of the increments.

Having an image on a screen, that can be clarified digitally has obvious advantages, and can help to reduce the subjective element of interpretation. However, this technique was not pursued to any depth, since the image is only a reflection of what exists on the thin section and it was felt that there are so many inherent problems with thin section analysis which arise from the limitations of the material rather than the way in which it is observed. This is not, of course, to detract form the value of computer image enhancement, which is an extremely useful tool in many kinds of analysis.

Confocal microscopy

In an attempt to establish the best method for viewing cementum layering, and to confirm that many of the difficulties encountered in incremental analysis are discrepancies in the material, not as a result of the technique employed to produce and analyse thin sections, confocal microscopy was attempted on some of the known aged sections. Boyde (pers. Comm. 1997) recommended this method. For a detailed description of confocal microscopy see Pawley (1995).

A confocal microscope is a modified light microscope that uses a laser beam and fluorescence to detect variations in mineral density of cementum. The specimen is viewed at X20 magnification. The microscope is able to focus on layers below the surface, and when focussed at a distance of 50 microns below the surface enables the internal structure of the cementum to be examined. The selected level of the specimen is then viewed as a black and white image on a VDU. I am grateful to Dr. Barry Brown, and to A. Boyde and S. Jones of the Department of Anatomy University College London who carried out this process.

A number of thin sections of the known aged sample were cleared in xylene and mounted under a cover slip in a thin DPX mix, and placed in an oven at 30C overnight prior to observation.

The following observations were made:

1. Bands and lines were identified in the same locations A to H which were observed under polarised light, and when present were very clearly defined.
2. Bands and lines could sometimes be followed along their lengths for several hundred microns.
3. The number of bands and lines varied from one location to the next, as observed under polarised light.
4. At some locations no bands or lines were visible.
5. The number of lines rarely coincided with the known age. Sometimes there were many fewer than the known age, and sometimes more.
6. Bands came in several levels of whiteness and darkness.
7. It was frequently difficult to decide where a line stopped and a band began.

Figure 46: Confocal microscopy of a Red deer aged 10 years and 8 months. Location H

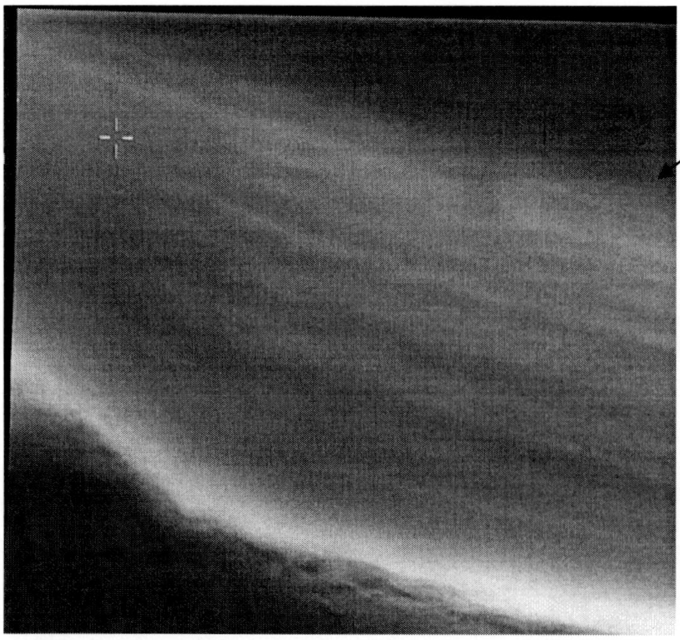

Bands and lines can be seen, but still cannot be related with confidence to age and season of death.

Figure 47: Confocal microscopy of a Red deer aged 13 years and 8 months. Location H

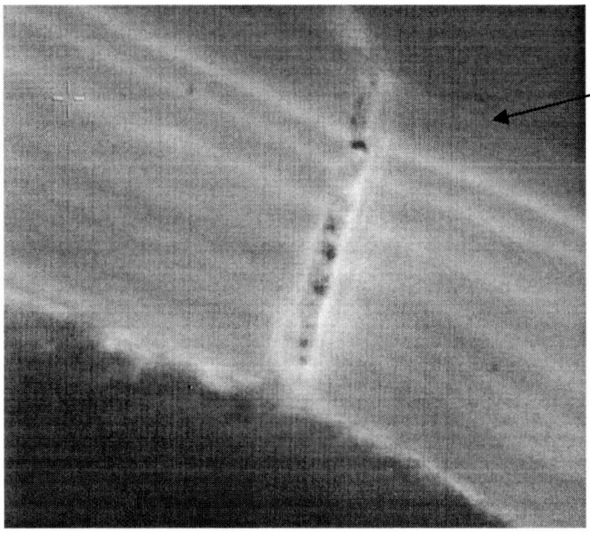

Figures 46 and 47 show images under confocal microscopy of two thin sections, from animals aged 10 years 8 months and 13 years 8 months respectively. Confocal microscopy gives an extremely clear picture of the bands and lines in cementum, and should be used as an alternative to polarised transmitted light microscopy. Although it makes the identification of bands and lines easier, it does not help in explaining what they represent, or in relating their number to the known age of the animal. This study confirms that, for red deer, treating the layers as annual structures and counting them to assess the age of the animal is inaccurate.

Chapter Five
Methods for Assessing Age using Wear of Teeth

The basis for ageing animals in a given population by tooth wear (or attrition) is that "if rate of wear in one homogeneous population is reasonably constant, then the extent of wear is a function of age" (Hillson 1986). In this chapter, the elements of a *scoring scheme* for age estimation based on tooth wear are described: the details of the scheme, and its statistical basis, are covered in the next chapter. The idea of a scoring scheme is that 'scores' are associated to various wear features on the teeth of the animal being studied and the total score of the jaw, obtained by adding together the scores for those wear features which are present, is correlated with the age of the animal.

The scheme presented here is based upon, and extends, a scheme devised by Brown and Chapman (1991): the principal extensions are the introduction of additional wear features, and a more formal statistical treatment to determine the scores which should be associated to each feature in order to optimise the accuracy of the scheme. The aim is to obtain the most accurate scheme possible, subject to the constraint that it be sufficiently simple to be implemented in the field without the benefit of expert training. In addition to being a worthy tool in its own right, the scheme provides a control for incremental analysis, where modern known aged material can be difficult to obtain.

In the archaeological context, age profiles can indicate hunting practice, with random kills being most likely the result of hunters picking the weaker animals, and cull patterns for domestic animals indicating herd management. They thus provide a valuable understanding of the socio-economic behaviour of prehistoric populations.

1. THE BASIS OF TOOTH WEAR

Eruption sequences

Before considering tooth wear itself, a discussion of tooth eruption sequences is necessary: eruption not only provides an accurate means of ageing young animals, but is itself essential for the accuracy of tooth wear analysis. Essentially tooth wear scores work as a system because teeth for a particular species always erupt in the same sequence, in the case of molars M1, M2 and M3. Therefore the scores for wear are steadily accumulative. Several authors have identified the ages at which red deer teeth erupt, or those at which they become functional: following Brown and Chapman (1991), these include Habermehl (1961), Mitchell (1967), Muller-Using (1971), von Raesfeld (1971), von Raesfeld and Vorreyer (1978), Wagenknecht (1981), and Drechser (1989). It is pointed out by Brown and Chapman that some of the discrepancies between these authors can be attributed to the fact that they do not make clear which event they are referring to, be it development or eruption.

I take the tooth eruption sequence of Brown and Chapman (1991) as being correct as they demonstrate a range of months in which each tooth erupts. Red deer tooth eruption proceeds according to the following sequence: the first molar erupts shortly after birth, the second follows, and then the third. Wear commences once a tooth has erupted fully, and meets the tooth or teeth on the opposing jaw - from this point on, a tooth wear scheme may be applied.

The dentition's of red deer are:

Deciduous I 0/3 c 1/1 pm 3/3
Permanent I 0/3 C 1/1 PM 3/3 M 3/3

Although eruption alone has been used for establishing age, this technique is only useful up to the age of about two years in deer (Brown and Chapman 1990), since after this point all of the teeth have erupted fully and are in wear. It has also been recognised that it may be possible to determine the season of death of younger animals from populations in which the ages at which eruption occurs are approximately uniform (references include Payne 1972, Carter 1997, Legge and Rowley-Conwy 1988).

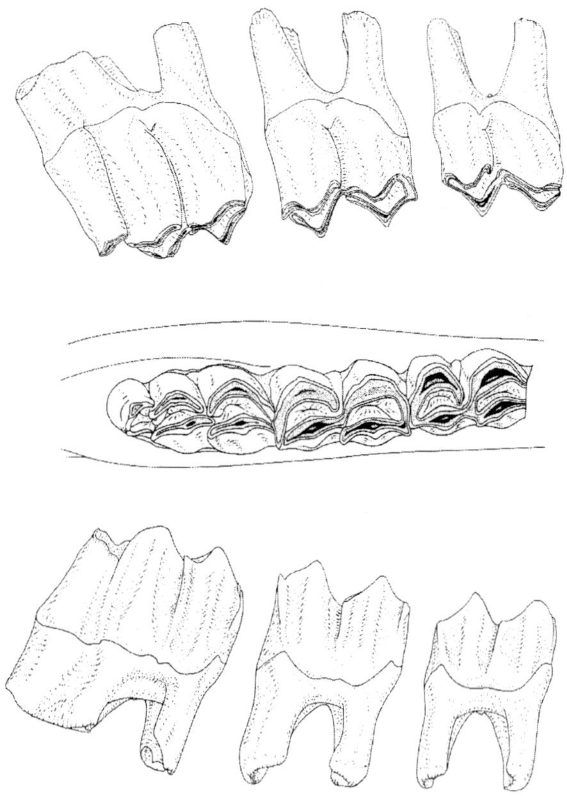

Figure 48. Red deer dentition

Tooth Wear

Given that ageing by means of eruption sequences is only appropriate to young animals, it is necessary to develop alternative techniques which can be applied when the teeth are in wear. Tooth wear occurs as grinding, mastication, and digestion takes place: both food contact and the taking in of abrasive particles from the ground play their part in this process. The occlusal surfaces of the teeth are subject to the earliest wear when the enamel on these surfaces is worn away. As the enamel is lost, dentine in the interior of the tooth becomes exposed, until eventually the occlusal surface becomes entirely dentine exposed. At the same time as the occlusal wear is taking place, wear is also occurring where the teeth of the same jaw are in contact with each other, which results in a loss of enamel at the area where the teeth meet, this is interstitial wear. Subsequent stages of tooth wear are described in more detail later in the chapter. As the tooth is worn down, adjustments are made in the jaw in order that the tooth is continually in wear (see the end of this chapter). The rate of wear itself depends on the age of the animal, being substantially faster in young animals. The idea behind all techniques for ageing by means of wear is to measure the extent of tooth wear, and to correlate this with the age of the animal: the differences between alternative schemes lie in the way in which wear is measured, and the means by which this is correlated with age. It is generally recognised that measurements of wear need only be taken on one half of a jaw, since there is very little difference in wear patterns between the left and right hand sides of the jaw in ungulates (Klein et al 1981). Very little work on wear is done on the upper jaw, but there is no reason why there shouldn't be.

Methods for measuring the extent of wear fall into two categories: those in which quantitative measurements of physical features of the teeth are made (most commonly crown height, although others are also used), and those which are based upon the presence or absence of qualitative features of the teeth. Although measurements of the former type might be supposed to be more objective than those of the latter, they are in fact subject to greater problems of interobserver reliability, and in addition tend to be less well correlated with age than the more qualitative measurements. Before proceeding to a description of the scoring scheme developed here, which is based on qualitative measurements (although quantitative measurements were also considered, and rejected on statistical grounds), a brief survey of ageing techniques based upon crown height and other measurements is appropriate.

Crown height measurements

Crown height measurements are generally taken on cheek (molar) teeth. The basic principle is the same as in all schemes based on tooth wear: that the teeth wear down over time, thus losing height as the animal ages. Hillson (1986) emphasises that ageing by crown height measurements commonly relies on a number of assumptions:

1. That the rate of wear is constant throughout an individual's life, and within a species
2. That the unworn crown height is the same for all animals of a given species.
3. That teeth erupt and come into wear at the same age for all animals of a species.
4. That the date of death corresponds to the end of a permanent tooth's functional life.

It should be added that these complications are often compounded by the fact that different researchers do not all use the same locations on the tooth for performing their measurements. Of course, several of these points apply equally to age assessment using scoring schemes based on qualitative features: however, it does appear that ageing by crown height is subject to substantial inaccuracies: individuals of the same age often show marked differences in crown height, particularly if they come from different environments (Lowe 1967, Klein et al. 1981). Klein et al. (1981) however claimed that, although crown height does not provide accurate ageing of individuals, it does permit animals to be assigned to relatively narrow age classes. This research contradicts this result.

Miller (1974) carried out one of the most detailed studies on Caribou. He measured the average height of the crown from the lowest point on the gum line to the highest point of the buccal ridge, in a population comprising both males and females. He then used multiple regression techniques to select the best combination of variables to be included in a formula to determine age, concluding that the best single indicator was obtained by adding the height of the p3 to that of the p4. Miller also went further than just using crown height measurements: he took 51 separate dental measurements for each tooth in the population. His conclusion was that eruption and replacement of mandibular teeth provided the greatest accuracy for animals up to 21 months, that root closure should be used for 2-3 year olds, and tooth height measurements for older animals. He also noted that males consistently show greater tooth wear than females.

Another interesting study, this time involving a sample of Fallow deer of known age, was carried out by Moore et al. (1995). They defined a tooth as having commenced eruption if any part of it was above the jawbone. The height was measured from the lowest point of the gum line (assuming the jaw had been defleshed, this would probably be from just above the jawbone) to the highest point of the crown, parallel to the long axis of the tooth. The first molars on both sides were measured from the enamel junction to the highest point on the mesial-buccal cusp, again parallel to the long axis. The Brown and Chapman scoring scheme was also applied to the same sample. Despite finding that different researchers could not reliably replicate crown height measurements, Moore et al believe that incisor height provides the most accurate method of ageing. Even if this is the case, it may not be as useful to archaeologists as to wildlife biologists, since incisors do not typically survive as well as molars in archaeological deposits. Another noteworthy observation is that they found that males initially have larger incisors than females, but that the teeth of males wear both faster and more regularly than those of females: they conclude that crown height measurements yield more accurate ageing for males than for females. Again, this has ramifications in archaeological applications, where it is not usually known which sex is being studied.

Factors affecting tooth wear: problems in ageing using tooth wear

A number of difficulties associated with the ageing of animals using tooth wear have already been mentioned, and it should be emphasised that the number of factors which affect the rate of tooth wear is sufficiently great that no scheme can do more than provide the approximate age (to within a few months) of the majority of animals; and that there will always be a few animals which, due to very unusual diet or health, will be subject to gross inaccuracies in age estimation (in fact, such 'outliers' are specifically taken into consideration in the statistical development of the scoring scheme). Even to provide this level of accuracy, there is no alternative to detailed analysis of modern populations of known age. In this section, the main factors which influence tooth wear, and the problems which they give rise to, are summarised.

1. Most obviously, tooth wear patterns and sequences are species-dependent, and schemes developed for one species cannot be applied to another, even to determine the relative ages of a number of individuals. This point was noted by Brown and Chapman (1990), who attempted to use existing scoring schemes devised for sheep and goats (Payne 1973), and for cattle (Grant 1982) to age the teeth of Fallow deer from Richmond park. Both of these methods were deemed unsuitable by the authors for assessing the age of Fallow deer.

2. The rate of tooth wear is affected by the quality of the diet of an animal, by the hardness of food, and by the type of ground from which they graze. It follows from this that ageing techniques developed for animals from a given environment may need to be modified to a greater or lesser extent when studying animals of the same species but from a different environment. Authors who have commented on this problem include Morris (1972), Perez-Barberia (1994), Chapman and Chapman (1975).

3. As has already been noted above, the rate of wear is typically different for males and females of the same species. The work of Miller (1974) and Moore et al. (1995) has already been discussed. Deniz and Payne (1982) noticed that the differences between male and female goats increased with age, so that the inaccuracies which would arise from a common scheme for both sexes would be greater for older animals. If the sex of the animal is known, then this problem is surmountable, but this is not always the case, particularly in archaeological work.

4. The rate of wear can be affected by the health of the animal: this factor is very difficult to take into consideration in age estimation.

5. Other factors which may affect the rate of wear are the height and depth of cusps and crevices, the area of the occlusal surface, the thickness and hardness of the enamel, and the overall morphology of the crown (Hillson 1986). These factors may be determined genetically. Kierdorf and Becher (1997) studied the degree of mineralization of enamel and coronal dentine of the first molar, and analysed the relationship between individual age, wear, and mineralization of the teeth. They concluded that the degree of mineralization has a decisive effect on dental wear, to which they attribute the high percentage of differences in molar attrition between animals of the same age.

6. In the archaeological context, it is possible that wear rates, and indeed eruption sequences, may vary between modern and ancient animals. In addition, some techniques may not be applicable to archaeological specimens (for example, measurements of height above the gum line).

7. A number of researchers have noted problems with both inter-observer and intra-observer reliability in tooth wear analysis: that is, that different researchers, and indeed a single researcher on different occasions, may measure the degree of tooth wear differently (Ewbank et al. 1964, Grant 1975, Payne 1973 in Aging and Sexing Animal Bones from Archaeological sites 1982). Often little work is done on checking the reliability of techniques. There is ample scope for subjectivity in comparing jaws with diagrams or photographs in order to assess wear stages (Grant 1975, Kierdorf and Becher 1997).

Comparison with incremental analysis

Tooth wear analysis is generally perceived to be less accurate than cementum incremental analysis (Miller 1974). Even if this were the case (a perception which is contested in this thesis), wear analysis has the advantage that it is quick, inexpensive, and does not require years of training and experience to be employed properly; moreover, it is a non-destructive technique, a benefit which is again of particular advantage in the archaeological context. Accurate ageing is also important to wildlife managers, who may not have a fully equipped laboratory at their disposal, or have the time or resources to send samples to professional laboratories for analysis.

Tooth wear and eruption have also been used as a control method for incremental analysis and vice-versa (Perez-Barberia 1994, Aitken 1975). It seems extraordinary that a quick, simple, and cheap method should be used to verify the accuracy of one which is slow, complex, and expensive: nevertheless, if this is to be done then the wear scheme must be as accurate as possible, and its accuracy must be known. As an example, Turner (1977) uses horn segments to age a collection of North American sheep, and then uses these age estimates to confirm the accuracy of cementum incremental analysis for the same animals.

2. STUDIES OF SUCCESSFUL AGEING USING TOOTH WEAR

In this section, some of the major work of other researchers on ageing animals using qualitative features of tooth wear is summarised. Work on archaeological samples, which is of particular relevance to this thesis, is described at the end of the section.

Deniz and Payne (1982), Payne (1987)

Deniz and Payne studied Turkish Angora goat in three flocks, amounting to approximately 750 animals of known age, and between 500 and 700 animals of unknown age. There were, however, limited numbers of males over 2½ years old and of females over 6-7 years old. They examined living animals, using incisor and left side cheek teeth eruption and wear: they identified nine age classes on the basis of the stage of dental eruption and the degree to which the enamel enfoldings were still visible on the occlusal surface (Davis 1987): these included the stage prior to dentine exposure, cusp dentine, isolation of infundibula, and loss of infundibula. The animals were examined ten times between November 1975 and November 1976. They claimed that the first two or three years of life differences between the animals born a year apart were so clear that wrongly numbered animals could be detected without the possibility of doubt or error. The timing of eruption showed little variability, although the usefulness of eruption in age estimation was limited, partly due to the length of the intervals between successive eruptions. As already mentioned above, they noted that differences between males and females seems to increase with age.

Grant (1982)

Grant observed stages of wear in an attempt to age domestic ungulates. She identified a number of 'tooth wear stages', starting when the enamel was worn and no dentine was exposed, going through to the latest stages when, in some cases, only the root remained in the jaw. She noted that the intervals between successive tooth wear stages did not represent equal intervals of time: however, by reference to tooth wear charts, it was possible to assign accurate wear stages of the deciduous fourth molar, the permanent fourth premolar, and the three permanent molars of cattle, sheep/goat, and pig mandibles. This allowed for determination of relative, but not absolute, ages of the animals studied.

Brown and Chapman (1990, 1991b)

Brown and Chapman undertook detailed analyses of fallow deer and red deer living in a protected environment, Richmond park, based on wear patterns (see Baxter Brown 1985, Chapman and Chapman 1970). They emphasised that the special nature of the population that they studied could lead to inaccuracies if their scheme was applied to other environments. For the analysis of red deer the number of animals available was insufficient for cohort analysis, and hence the males and females were grouped together.[1] In their initial studies, Brown and Chapman made use of the following sequential changes in tooth wear:

After Brown and Chapman 1990.

Type of wear	Score given
Enamel wear on slopes	1
Dentine wear on slopes	2
Central eye between slopes	1
Dentine links between lingual and buccal cusps:	
i) mesial ridge	1
ii) between the mesial and distal cusps	1
iii) distal ridge	1
Dentine links between mesial and distal cusps:	
i) lingual aspect	1
ii) buccal aspect	1
Third molar hypoconulid dentine exposed	
i) lingual aspect	1
ii) buccal aspect	1
iii) distal linking of (I) and (ii)	1
iv) link with lingual cusp	1
v) link with buccal cusp	1
vi) link between lingual and buccal cusps	1
All infundibulum worn away	1
Black staining of exposed dentine	1

Table 7: Scoring elements in the Brown and Chapman scheme (Brown and Chapman 1990)

The current author tested the Brown-Chapman scheme on a known aged sample of 70 Scottish Red deer mandibles which were kindly donated by the Deer Commission for Scotland. It was noted that, although the scheme was accurate for younger animals, it was subject to inaccuracies of several years when applied to the older animals (over five years). It was in an attempt to extend the Brown-Chapman scheme to older animals that the scoring scheme described later in this chapter was devised. I am very grateful to Norma Chapman for her support in the extension of this scheme. The Brown-Chapman scheme was also applied by Moore et al. (1995) to Irish Fallow deer: they found that the scheme aged over 75% of the animals aged between 4 and 35 months accurately, but that one was aged incorrectly by 3 years, and that the older animals were much less accurately aged.

Kierdorf and Becher (1997)

Kierdorf and Becher studied a population of Red deer: in an attempt to eliminate problems of inter-observer reliability, they carried out dentine width measurements on the mesiobuccal cusp of the M1 to the nearest

[1] Noting this point Brown took the new scoring scheme to Rum and applied it to males and females whom can be studied separately. Results in press.

millimetre. As already mentioned, they also studied the degree of mineralization of enamel and coronal dentine, and correlated this with age and wear. They concluded that the Brown-Chapman system provided more accurate results, and suggested that the increased variation in wear score for older animals in the Brown-Chapman scheme reflected difference in wear resistance due to variations in enamel mineralization.

Other work

As well as the work cited above, other tooth wear analysis has been successfully applied, and should be examined by any researcher wishing to use tooth wear analysis for ageing animals.
For cattle see (Brown et al.1960), Red deer (Ratcliffe 1987, aimed at wildlife managers who need a quick and simple way to get a rough approximation of age), humans (Molleson and Cohen 1990), Mule deer (Robinette et al. 1957), Fallow deer (Chapman and Chapman 1970, 1975), Roe deer (Aitken 1975, Legge and Rowley-Conwy 1988).

Archaeological applications of tooth wear analysis
As has already been discussed, there are particular problems associated with attempting to apply eruption and wear sequences to archaeological fauna: nevertheless, this has been attempted by a number of researchers in an attempt to establish both age and season of death of animals on an archaeological site. Legge and Rowley-Conwy (1988) successfully employed eruption sequences to age Roe deer from Star Carr, concluding that all of the animals were killed in the late spring and summer. They also considered crown height measurements in an attempt to establish seasonality from Roe deer whose teeth were fully erupted and in wear: based on the observation that many teeth had the same height, they deduced that there was a restricted culling time.

Other authors have reported more problems in applying wear schemes to archaeological material. Levitan (1982) used both Grant's and Payne's scoring system on a random sample of 200 mandibles from the Romano-British temple complex at West Hill, Uley, Gloucestershire. Errors were made when the teeth were not clean, and Grant's method gave rise to problems when a wear pattern did not fit into a single stage, but appeared to combine characteristics of two. Hamington (1982) studied approximately 170 Iron Age sheep mandibles from Ashville Trading Estate, Oxfordshire. Different workers gave different results, using both tooth eruption and wear sequences.

3. A NEW SCORING SCHEME FOR RED DEER

Motivation and aims
As mentioned above, the author applied the Brown-Chapman scoring scheme to a population of deer donated by the Deer Commission for Scotland. The deer were of known age, having been tagged at birth, and ranged in age from 5 months to 16 years, with every year being represented 2 to 3 times; males and females were equally represented, and the animals were from natural environments, more likely to be reflective of archaeological specimens. I would like to thank the Deer Commission for Scotland and in particular, Colin McLean who made this study possible.

When the scheme had been applied, it became clear that errors were occurring, primarily in animals over 5 years old, leading to both underestimates and overestimates of age. It was therefore desirable to modify and extend the scheme, in such a way as to provide better age estimation for older animals. I am grateful to Barry Brown for his advice and support in the development of the extended scheme. In order to achieve an accurate extension of the scheme, new wear features were introduced in order to match older age classes. All of the features can be scored independently, which allows for reliability testing between teeth scored and between different researchers - any differences in scores recorded can be identified and re-evaluated. The relative weights to be assigned to each of the wear features were optimised using statistical techniques. I am appreciative of the specialist advice in this area provided by David Downham and Toby Hall. Once the scheme had been devised, both its accuracy and the reliability with which the same and different examiners could replicate the same results were studied in detail: accuracy and reliability were both found to be very good.
In the remainder of this chapter, the different wear features, which are assumed to develop progressively with age, are introduced. In the next chapter, the statistical analysis which yields the final scoring scheme is described. This is followed by an analysis of accuracy and reliability.

The first step, then, was to identify the 'scoring elements' that would be used in the scoring scheme: that is, features of a tooth that develops progressively as the animal ages. This was achieved by laying out and studying in detail a large known age sample, covering the whole spectrum from 5 months to over 16 years old. A total of 16 different scoring elements for each molar were identified (with one additional element relating to the hypoconulid of the third molar), only some of which, namely have been used in previous attempts to estimate age from wear (see above). The scoring elements fall into two categories: *discrete* elements, which can take on only whole number values (for example, the number of mesial-distal links, or the number of lingual crests lost), and *continuous* elements, which can take on any value (for example, the crown heights and tooth width). It is clear that discrete elements can in general be measured more rapidly and reliably than continuous ones.

Only molariform teeth were used in this scoring scheme. Initially, in an attempt to obtain results as accurate as possible, incisors were also included in the study. However, it was found that they added no value to the overall age determination, and complicated the examination procedure. It was therefore decided that they should not be included in the scheme.

The scoring elements identified were the following: each is described in more detail below:

1. Cuspal wear of enamel.
2. Cuspal wear of dentine.
3. Exposure of dentine continuously between a) Lingual and buccal cusps; b) anterior and posterior cusps; and c) wear of the hypoconulid of the third molar.
4. Loss of the infundibulum of the hypoconulid.
5. Conversion of the infundibula from clefts to pits enclosed by enamel and surrounded by dentine.
6. Narrowing of the mouths of the infundibula.
7. Roots visible above bone of alveolar crest.
8. Enamel contact points between the teeth lost.
9. Acute angle of cusp tips worn to an obtuse angle on a) the buccal side and b) the lingual side.
10. Loss of the vertical lingual crests of the crown.
11. Posterior Dentine width
12. Tooth width.
13. Lingual crown height.
14. Buccal crown height.

These scores are cumulative. for example, if an infundibulum is lost, and therefore scores one, this would be added to the score already counted as the maximum score possible for infundibulum narrowing.

Scoring scheme elements

The scoring scheme was developed by examining a number of features and assessing their presence or absence on a large sample of known aged jaws. A detailed statistical examination was then carried out to determine what weight should be assigned to each feature in order to arrive at the most accurate possible estimate of age. A number of the features were assigned weight zero, which means that in practice they do not need to be considered when applying the scoring scheme. All features examined are detailed below. A summary of the features used in the final scheme is given at the end of this section.

Cuspal enamel wear and exposure of dentine

Wear of the cuspal enamel begins as soon as the teeth have erupted sufficiently to bring the teeth of opposing jaws into contact. The enamel of the cusp is worn on the anterior and posterior slopes of the anterior lingual and buccal cusps, followed by the posterior lingual and buccal cusps. The enamel on these slopes is quite thin and wears quite rapidly.

When the scoring sheme was being developed, and in the initial Brown and Chapman scheme (1990), the enamel worn was given a score of one for each cusp slope. However, because the enamel is worn so quickly, it became unnecessary to use this element in the final scheme. Statistically this element made no difference to the final score.

Once the enamel has been worn away on the cuspal slopes, the dentine becomes exposed. The dentine is identified as a yellow colour, which turns brown over time.

Dentine links

As wear of the cusps increases through time, more dentine is exposed so that it is seen as being continuous between a) the lingual and buccal cusps and b) the paired lingual cusps and the paired buccal cusps.

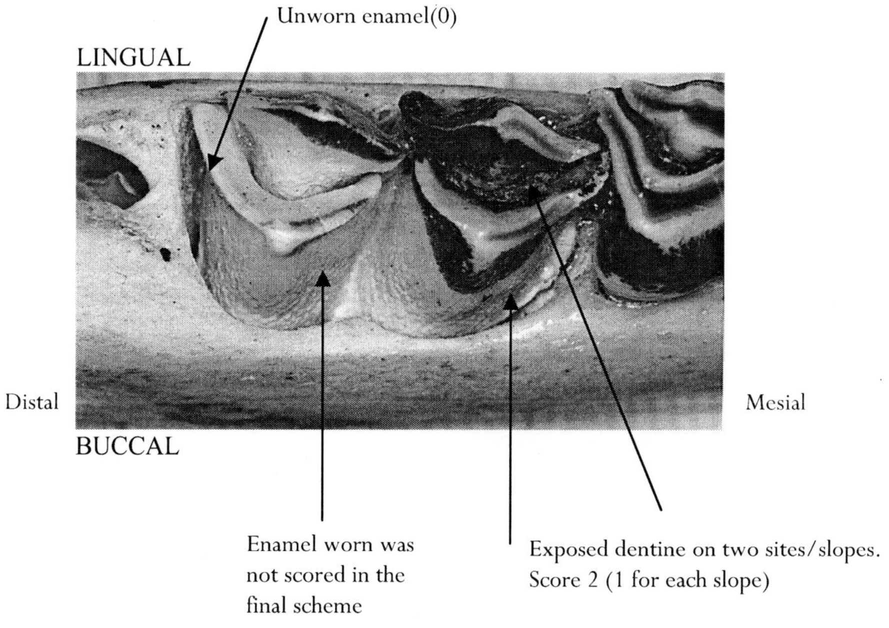

Figure 49: Enamel wear, and the beginning of dentine exposed.

Figure 50: Dentine exposed six slopes of the M2

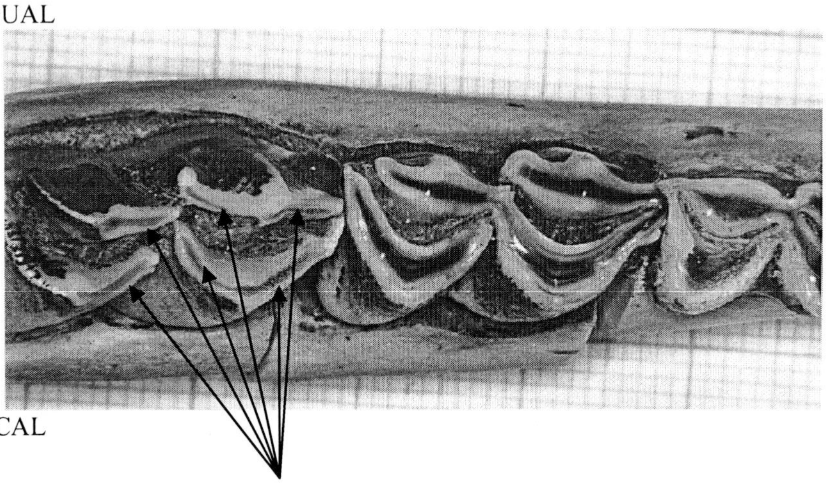

Figure 51: Dentine links on one site of an M1 (buccal to lingual)

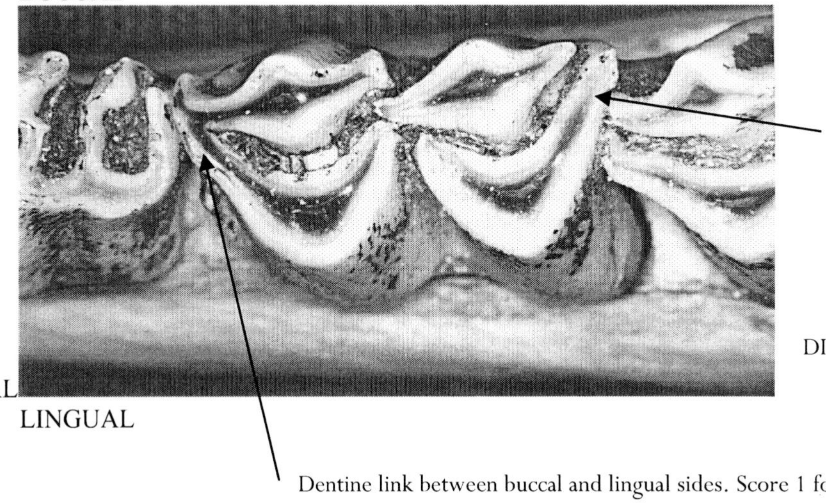

Figure 52: Dentine links on M1 in one site (mesial to distal) and two sites (lingual to buccal)

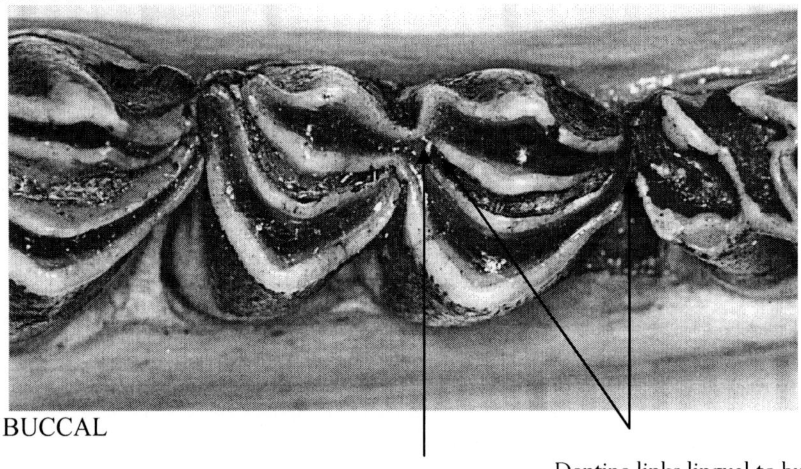

Figure 53: Dentine links on M1 lingual to buccal in three sites

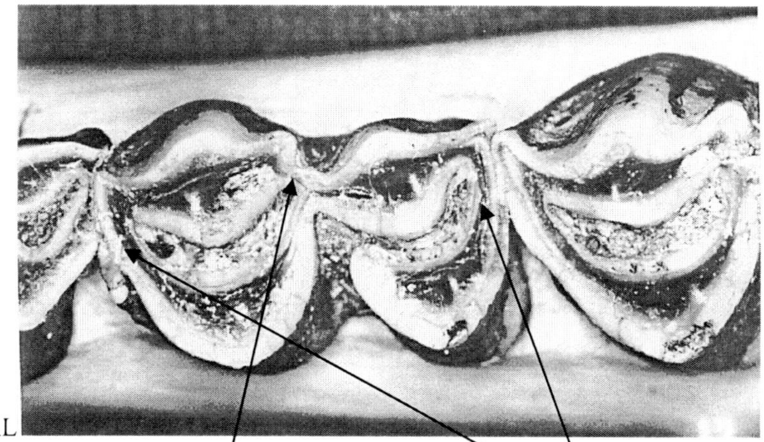

Figure 54: Dentine links mesial to distal and lingual to buccal on an older animal.

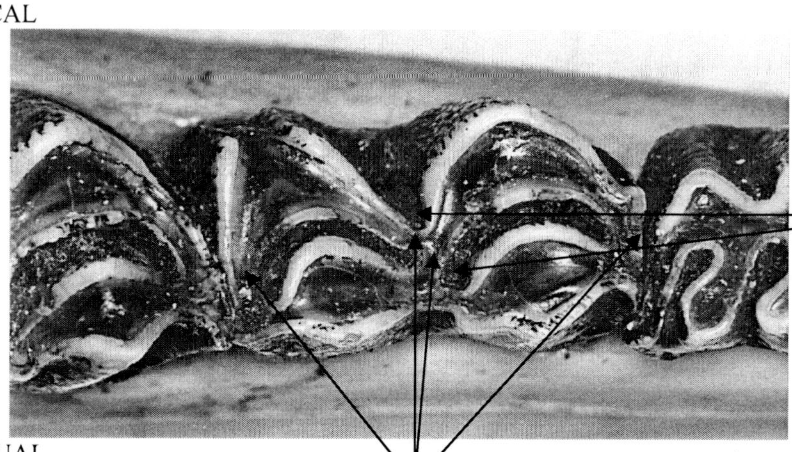
BUCCAL
MESIAL
Dentine links mesial to distal Score 3 for each link. Two links give a score of 6 for mesial distal links for this tooth.
DISTAL
LINGUAL
Dentine links lingual to buccal score for each link. Four links on this tooth score 4 for these links for this tooth.

The hypoconulid of the third molar forms four links between its lingual and buccal sides and to the posterior cusps of the third molar.

Figure 55: The hypoconulid and the third molar, dentine links

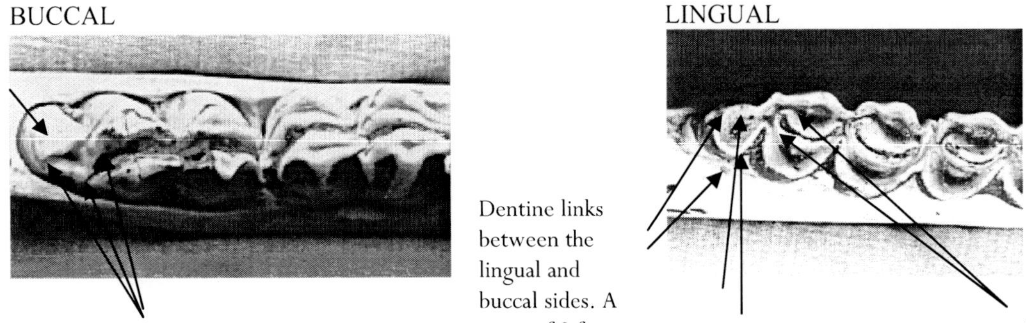

In the initial examination of the scheme, the infundibulum of the hypoconulid becoming completely surrounded by exposed dentine and eventually lost was scored. However statistically this made no difference to the overall age and was therefore not incorporated into the final scheme.

Infundibulum closing

The three molars each have two infundibula located between their lingual and buccal cusps. The third molar has a small additional infundibulum on the posterior hypoconulid which is analysed separately (see above). Initially when the tooth erupts, before any wear has taken place, the infundibula appear as simple clefts between the lingual and buccal cusps, which may open on the anterior, lingual, buccal or posterior surface of the tooth. With the wearing away of the cusps, the infundibula become bow shaped pits with enamel lips surrounded by exposed dentine.

Figure 56: Infundibulum closing on two sites of the M2

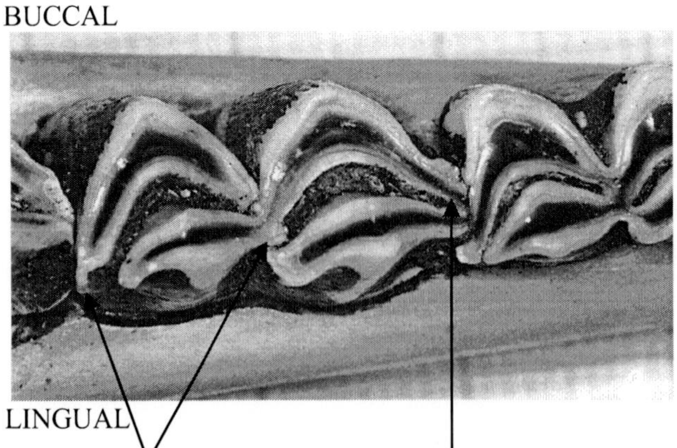

Figure 57: Infundibulum narrowing on two sites of the M1

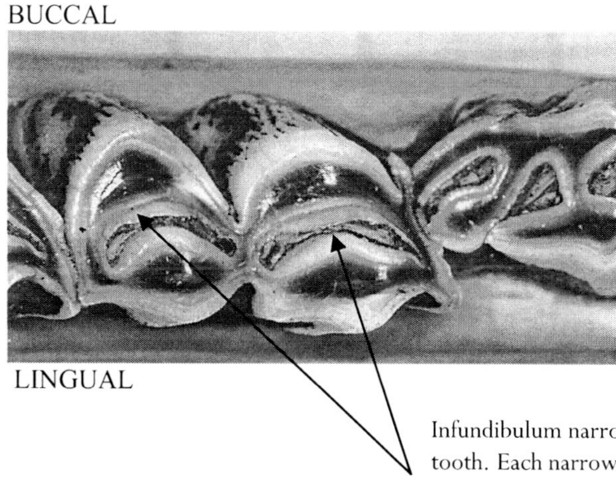

Infundibulum narrowing

Once the infundibula are exposed by a continuous layer of enamel, they are seen as separate entities surrounded by dentine. With wear their enamel bow-shaped lips become reduced in size until their opposing edges approximate towards each other. In the final wear stages the infundibula are seen as small slits and in the very last stages become small pinpoints of enamel.

Figure 58: Infundibulum narrowing on six sites of the M1

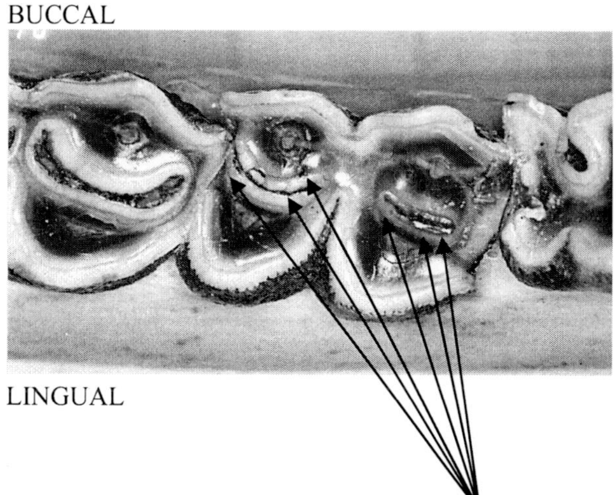

Figure 59: Infundibulum lost on the M1

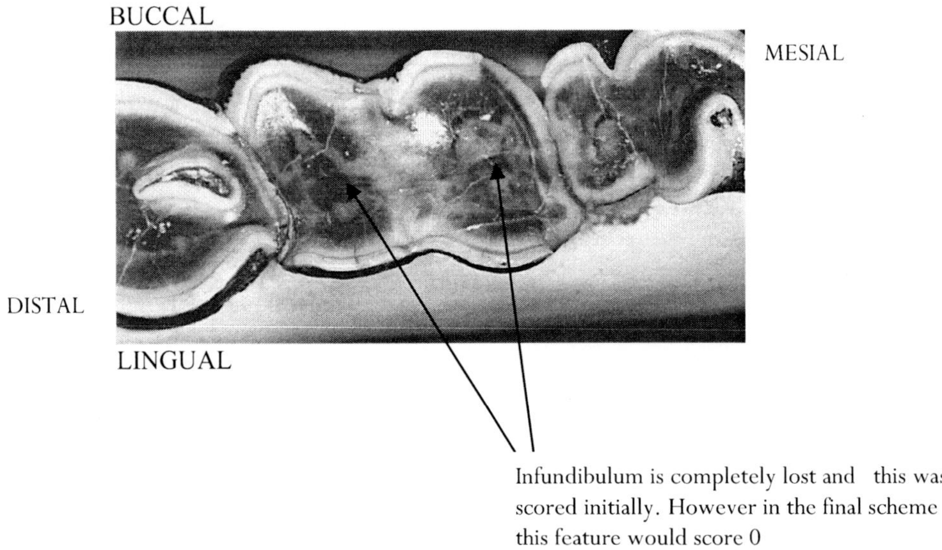

Roots visible above the bone of the alveolar crest.

Teeth erupt continually throughout life and eventually roots appear above the edge of the bone of the alveolar crest. This keeps the tooth in wear.

Figure 60: Root visible above the alveolar crest lingual and buccal views

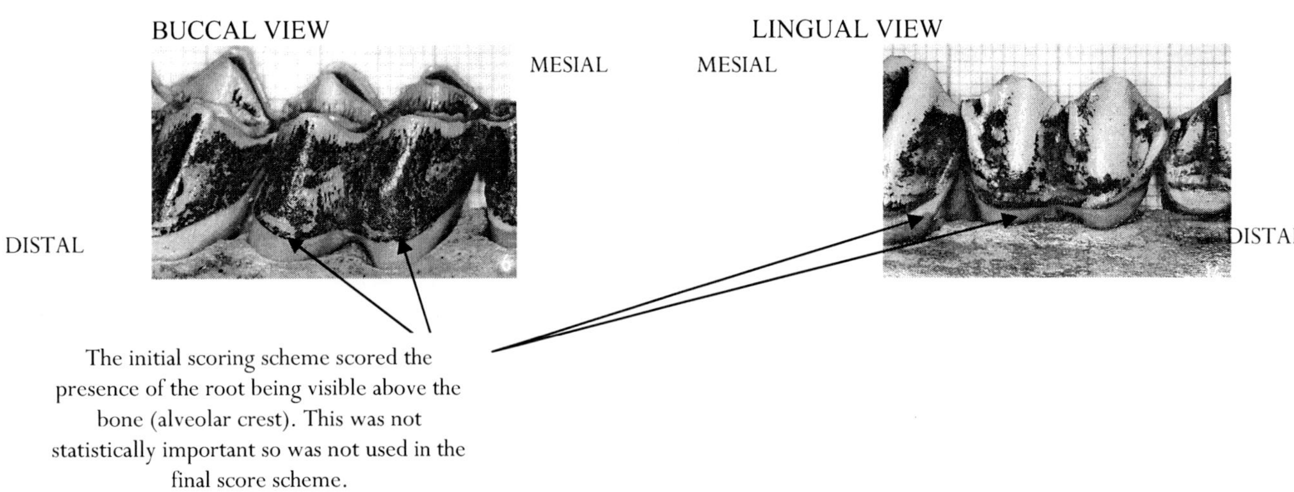

Figure 61: Contact enamel lost on both sides of the M1

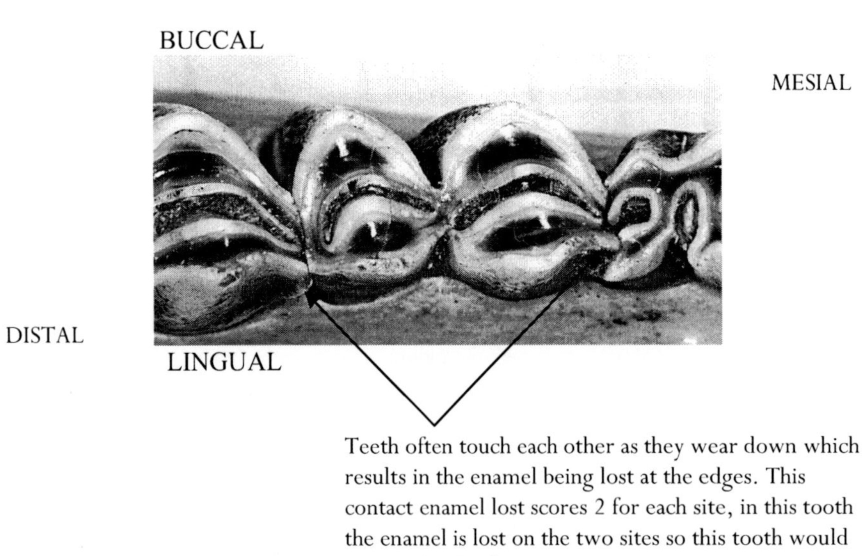

Acute to obtuse angles

The angles of the cusp on both the lingual and buccal sides were examined. Statistically it was only the lingual side that was significant. Therefore in the final scheme it is the lingual side that was given a score.

Figure 62: Cusp wearing from being triangular (acute) to obtuse angle on the lingual side of M1

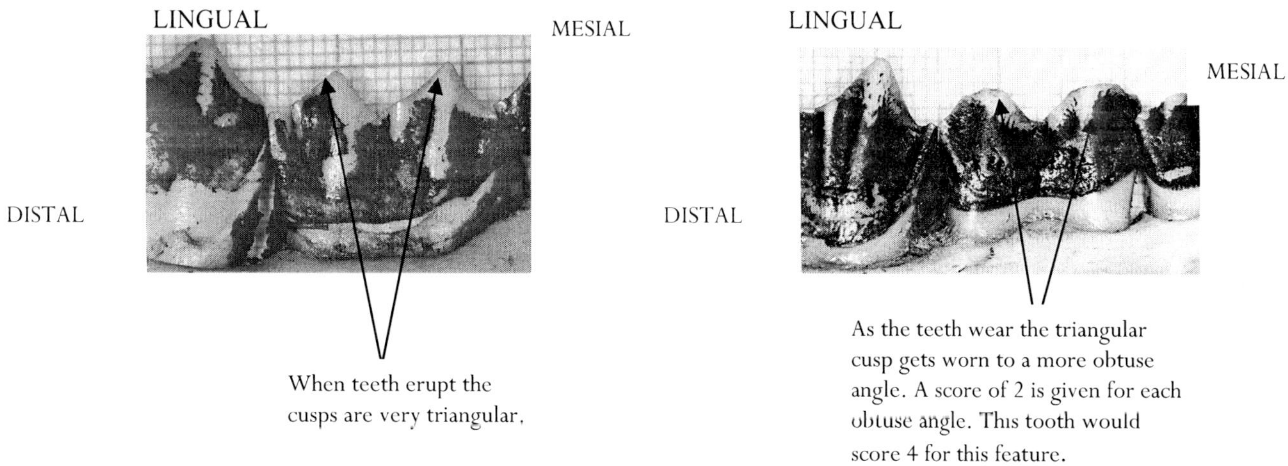

Lingual crests lost

The folds, vertical crests of enamel which extend from the cusp edge to a third or less of the crown height and ridges, which form the main bulk of the cusps extending from the cusp edge to the cervical margin, are well defined on newly erupted teeth.

Figure 63: Lingual crests lost on buccal side of M1

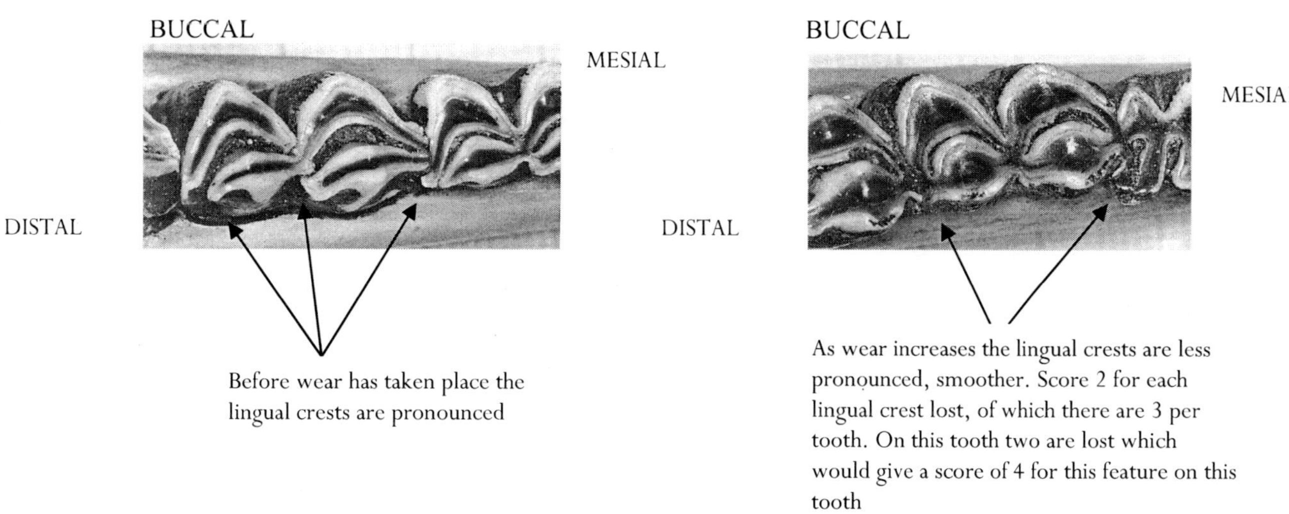

Figure 64: Lingual crests lost on M1

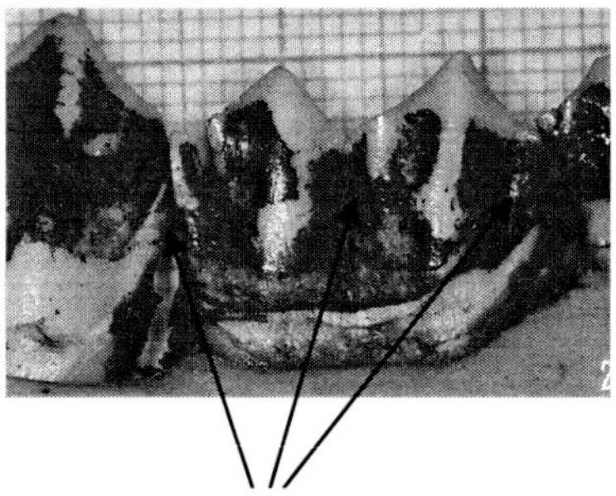

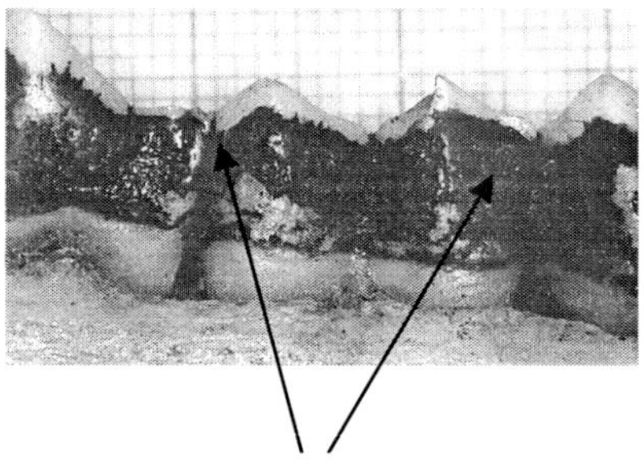

The scores outlined above are cumulative: for example, if an infundibulum is lost, and therefore scores one, this would be added to the score already counted as the maximum score possible for infundibulum narrowing.

A summary of the features used to score, with the complete score is provided below.

4. STEP BY ST

Taking one feature at a time, but scoring that feature for the whole jaw, the aim is to arrive at an estimated age for the animal. The photographs below represent one animal. Illustrations at the end of this section may help to clarify some of the scoring elements described below.

a) Dentine exposed on cuspal slopes.

Figure 65: Step by Step guide to scoring jaws

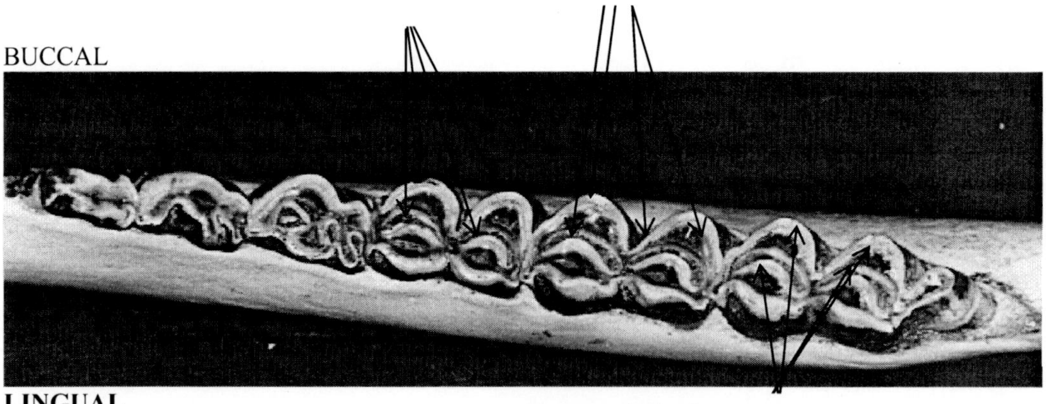

The total score for dentine exposed on this jaw is 4 + 4 + 4 = 12

b) Dentine links lingual to buccal

Dentine links lingual to buccal, score 1 for each link. On this M1 there are four links. The score for the M1 is 4

Dentine links lingual to buccal, score 1 for each link. On this M2 there are four links. The score for this M2 is 4.

BUCCAL

MESIAL

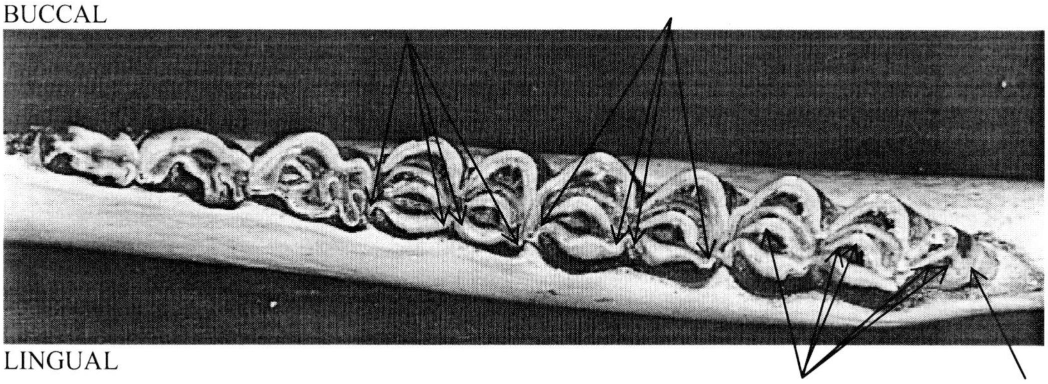

DISTAL

LINGUAL

Dentine links lingual to buccal. Score 1 for each link. On this M3 there are six links due to the hypoconulid. The score for this M3 is 6.

Total score for links lingual to buccal on this jaw is 4 + 4 + 6 = 14

c) Dentine links mesial to distal

Dentine links mesial to distal. Score 3 for each link. On this M1 there are two links. The score for this M1 is 6.

Dentine links mesial to distal. Score 3 for each link. On this M2 there are two links. The score for this M1 is 6.

BUCCAL

MESIAL

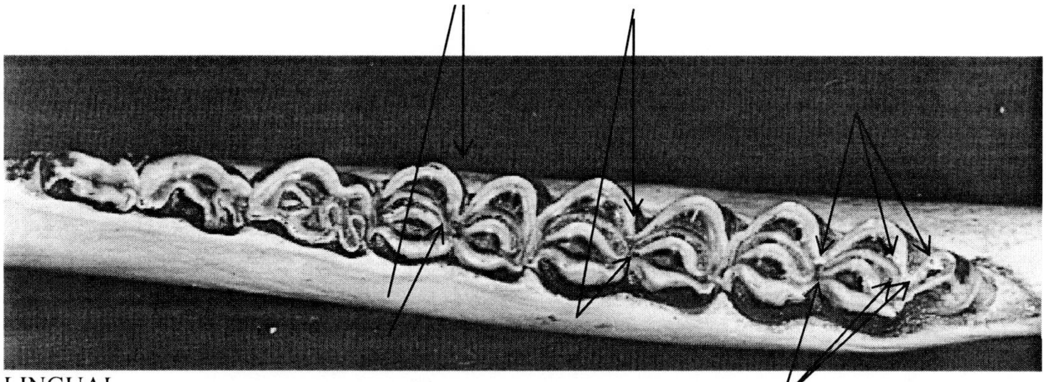

DISTAL

LINGUAL

Dentine links mesial to distal. Score 3 for each link. On this M3 there are six links. Two links between the anterior and posterior cusps, two between the cusp and the hypoconulid and two for the links on the lingual and buccal sides of the hypoconulid. The score for this M3 is 18.

Total score for links mesial to distal on this jaw is 6 + 6 + 18 = 30

d) Infundibulum closing

The infundibulum is closing when the ends are surrounded by dentine.

The infundibulum is closing (surrounded by dentine) on all four ends of the infundibulum. Score 3 for each site. This M1 scores 12 for this feature.

The infundibulum is closing (surrounded by dentine) on all four ends of the infundibulum. Score 3 for each site. This M2 scores 12 for this feature.

BUCCAL

MESIAL

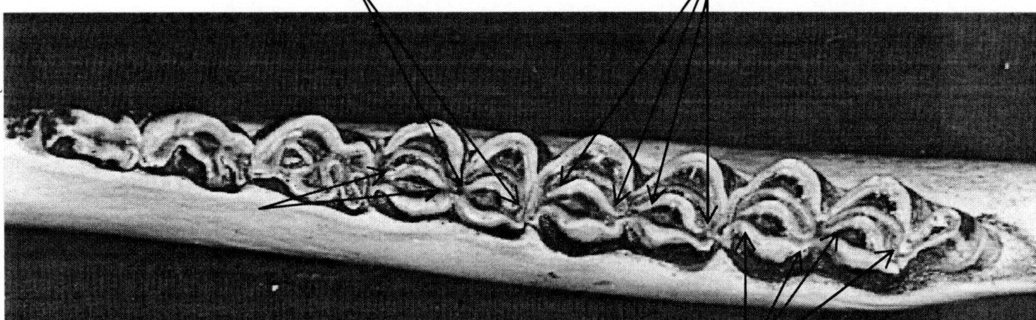

LINGUAL

DISTAL

The infundibulum is closing (surrounded by dentine) on all four ends of the infundibulum. Score 3 for each site. This M3 scores 12 for this feature.

Total score for the infundibulum closing on this jaw is 12 + 12 + 12 = 36

e) Infundibulum narrowing

Once the infundibula are surrounded by dentine and as wear progresses the lips of the infundibulum move towards each other causing a narrowing of the infundibulum. This occurs on three sites per cusp of each molar – at either end of the infundibulum and in the middle. On the whole, the middle of the infundibulum narrows first.

Infundibulum narrowing in two sites on this M2. Score 2 for each site. This M2 has a total score of 4.

Infundibulum narrowing in two sites on this M1. Score 2 for each site. This M1 has a total score of 4.

BUCCAL

MESIAL

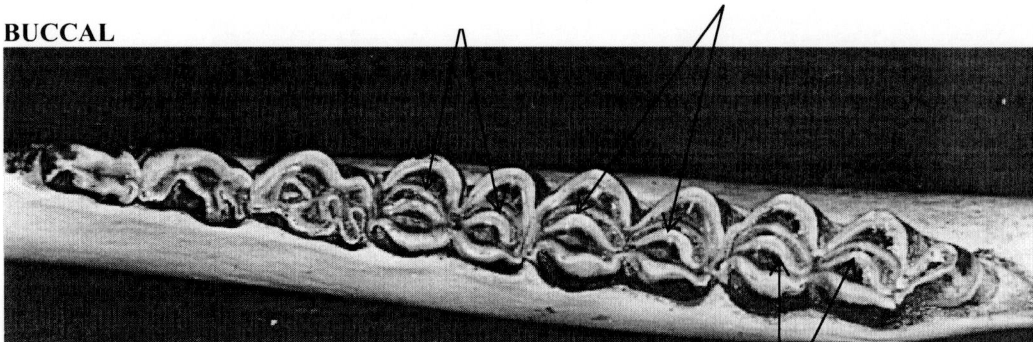

DISTAL

LINGUAL

Infundibulum narrowing in two sites on this M3. Score 2 for each site. This M3 has a total score of 4.

Total score for the infundibulum narrow

f) Contact enamel lost

The enamel between the teeth has been worn away in this area. For contact enamel lost score 2 for each point lost. For this M1 the contact enamel has been lost in two sites. This tooth scores 4.

MESIAL

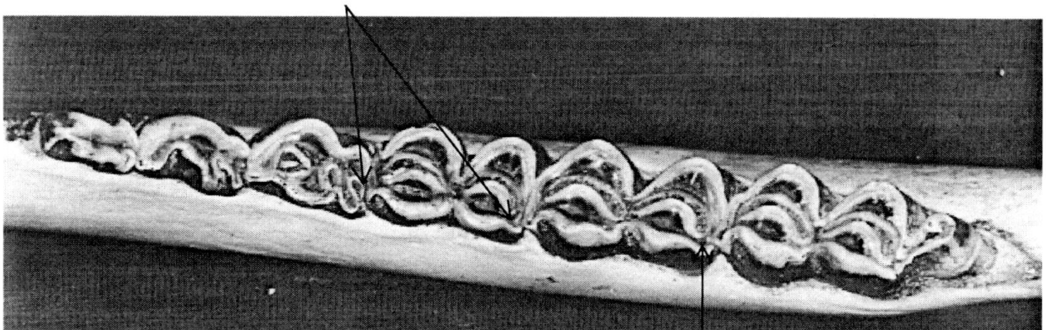

DISTAL

For this M2 the contact enamel has been lost in one site. This tooth scores 2.

There is no contact enamel lost on the M3, so score 0.

Total score for contact enamel lost on this jaw is 4+ 2+ 0= 6

g) Lingual acute angle lost

Lingual cusps have lost the triangular tip through wear. Both cusps have lost the acute angle. Score 2 for each acute angle lost. This M1 scores 4.

Lingual cusps have slightly lost the triangular tip through wear, but they have not become an acute angle yet. This M2 scores 0.

MESIAL

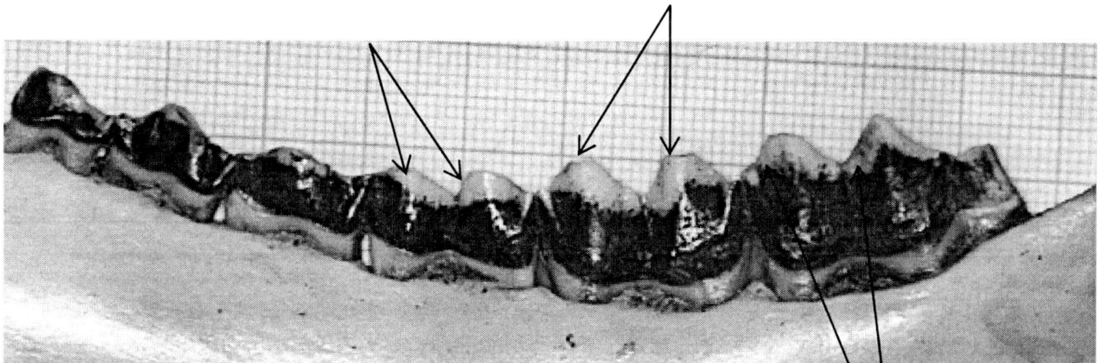

DISTAL

M3 has not lost the acute angle on either cusp. Score 0.

Total score for lingual acute angle lost on this jaw is 4+ 0+ 0 = 4

h) Lingual crests lost

BUCCAL

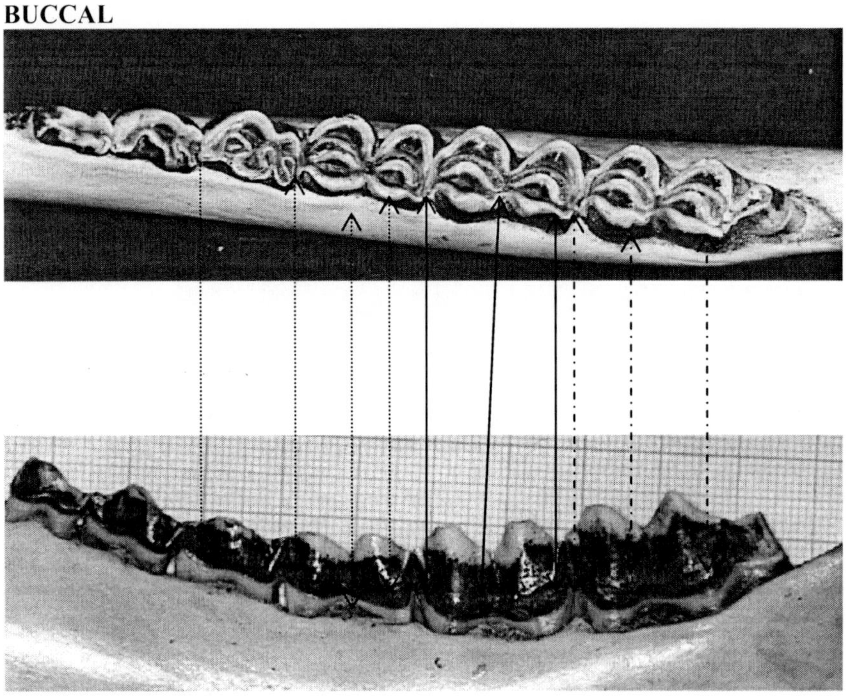

M1 has lost only the middle crest (it is smooth). Score 2 for each crest lost. This tooth scores 2.

The M2 and M3 have all their lingual crests. Score 0.

The scores are cumulative and should therefore be added together to give an approximation to the total age in months of the animal. Once the scores for each of the three molars have been summed, a constant value of 3 should be added to the total score – the reasons for the addition of this constant are given in detail in Chapter 6.

The total score for this jaw is therefore 119: thus the estimated age is 119 months (9 years 11 months).

Step by step illustrated guide for identification of sequential wear of Red deer teeth
Illustrations by Sandra Doyle

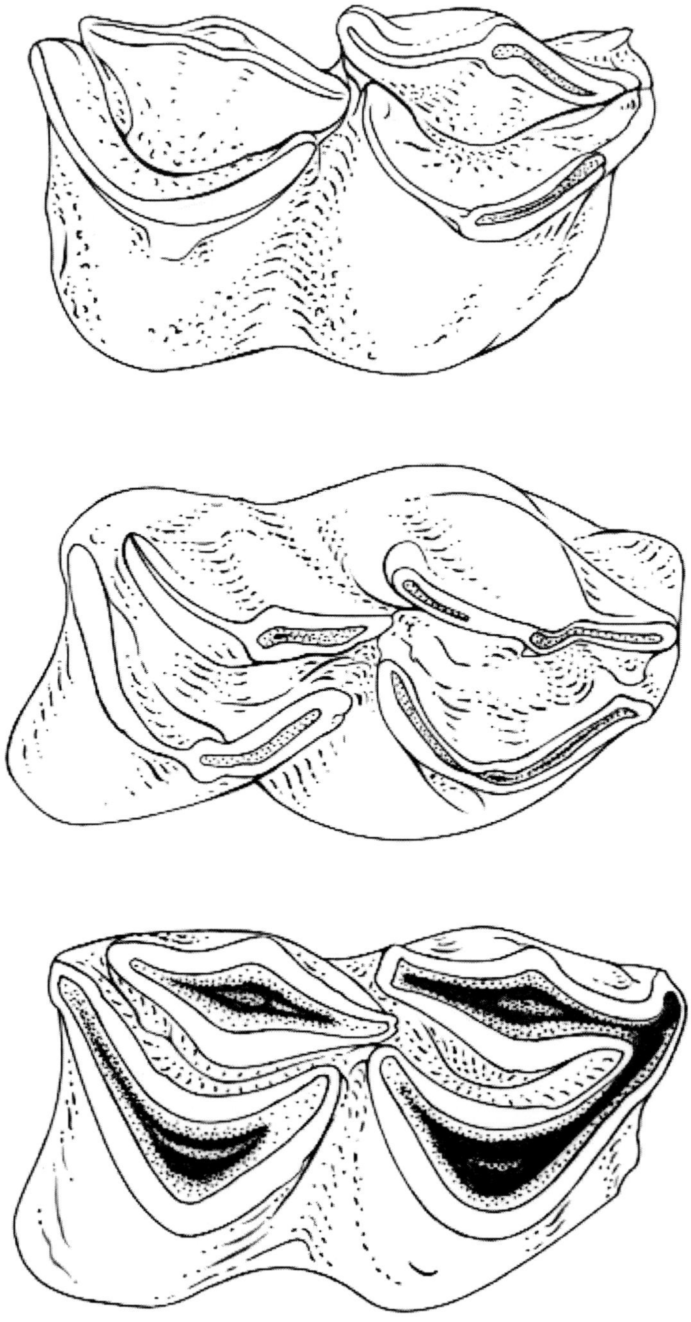

Illustration 1
Areas of exposed Dentine

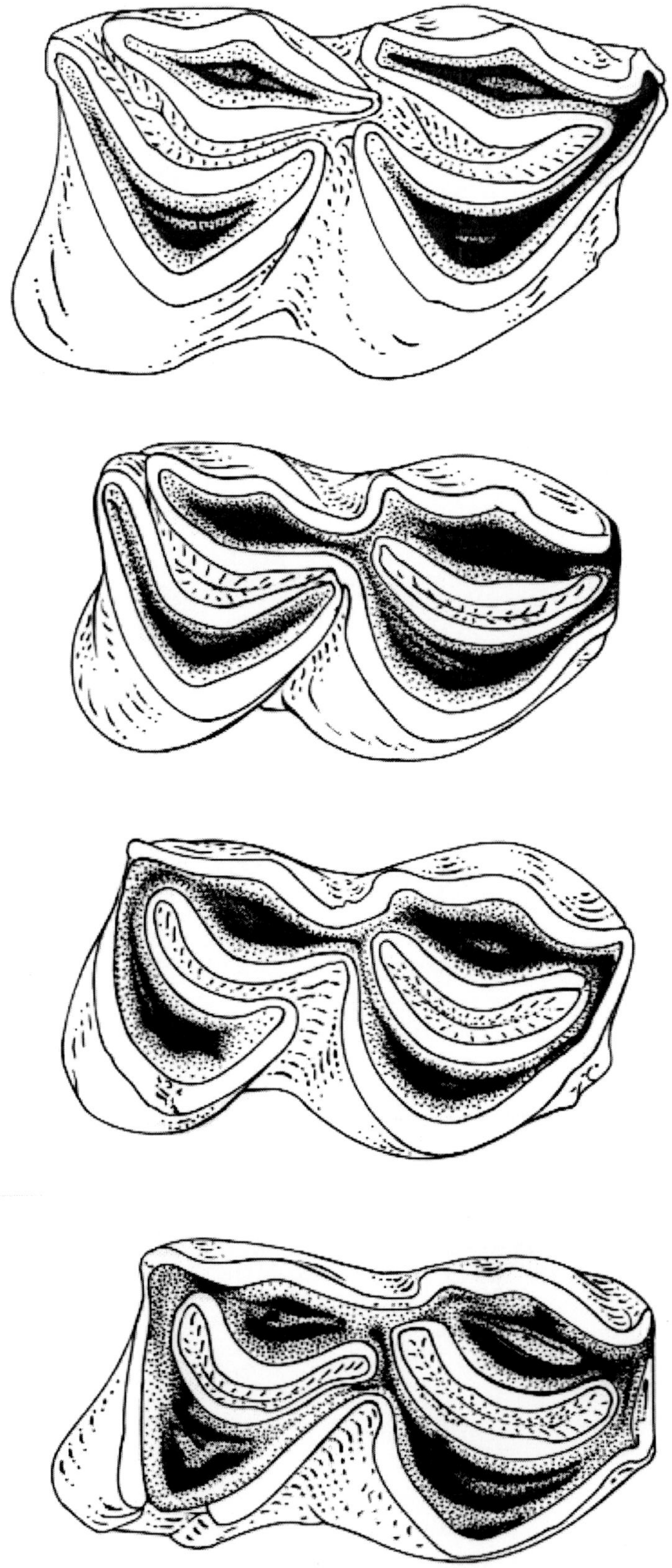

Illustration 2
Continuous exposure of dentine between lingual and buccal cusps, and between mesial and distal cusps

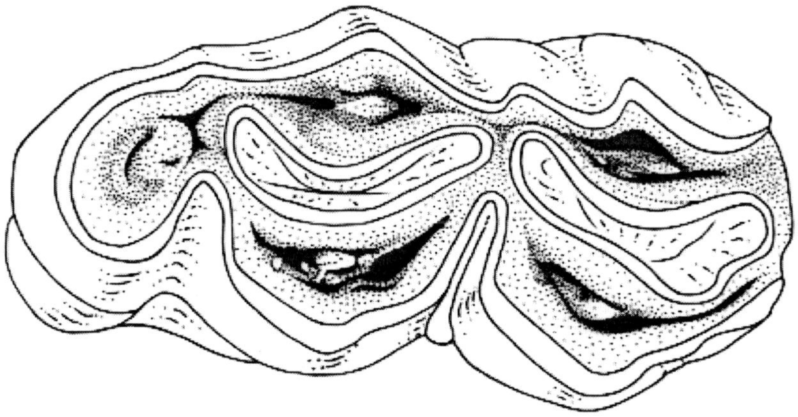

Illustration 3
Continuous dentine links including the hypoconulid

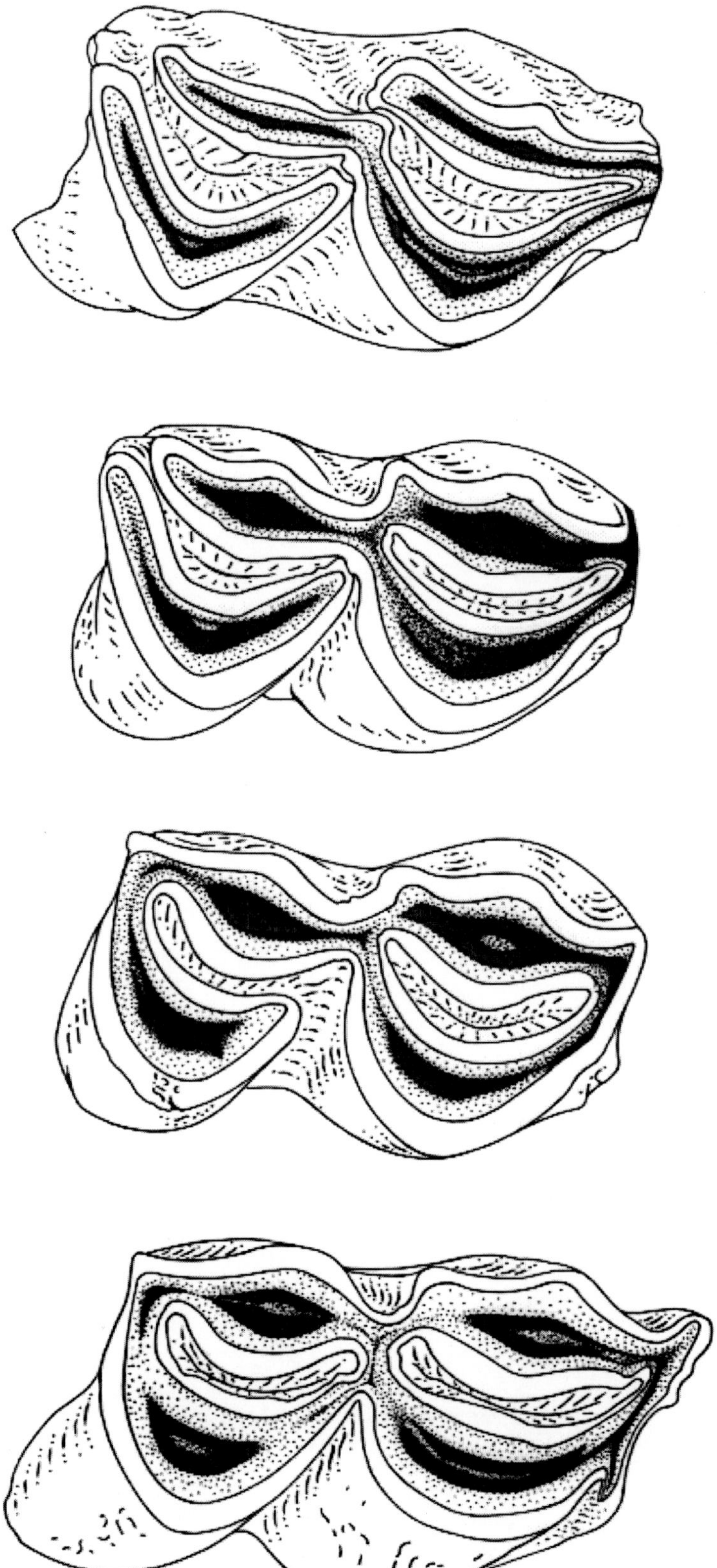

Illustration 4
Conversion of the infundibula from clefts to pits, which are enclosed by enamel surrounded by exposed dentine

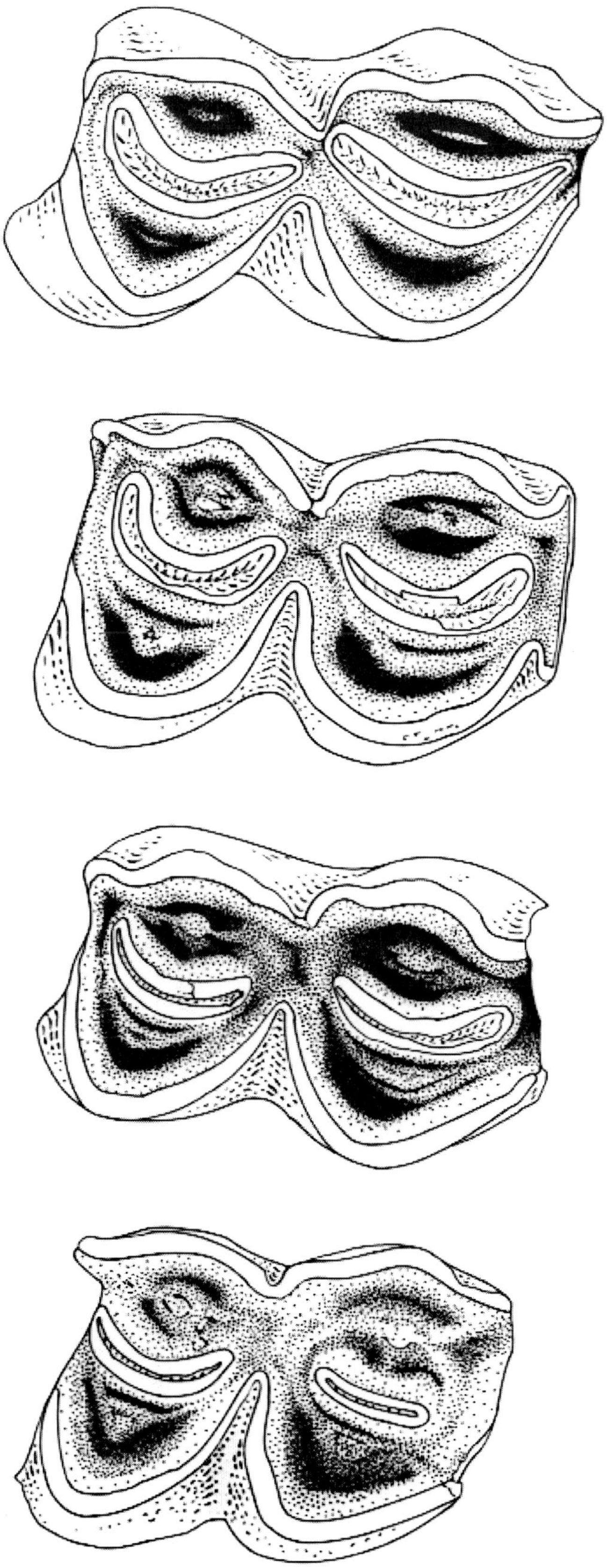

Illustration 5
Narrowing of the infundibula

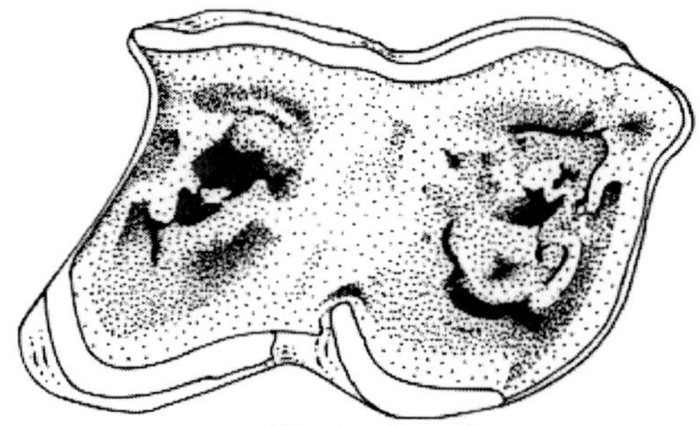

Illustration 6
Loss of the infundibula

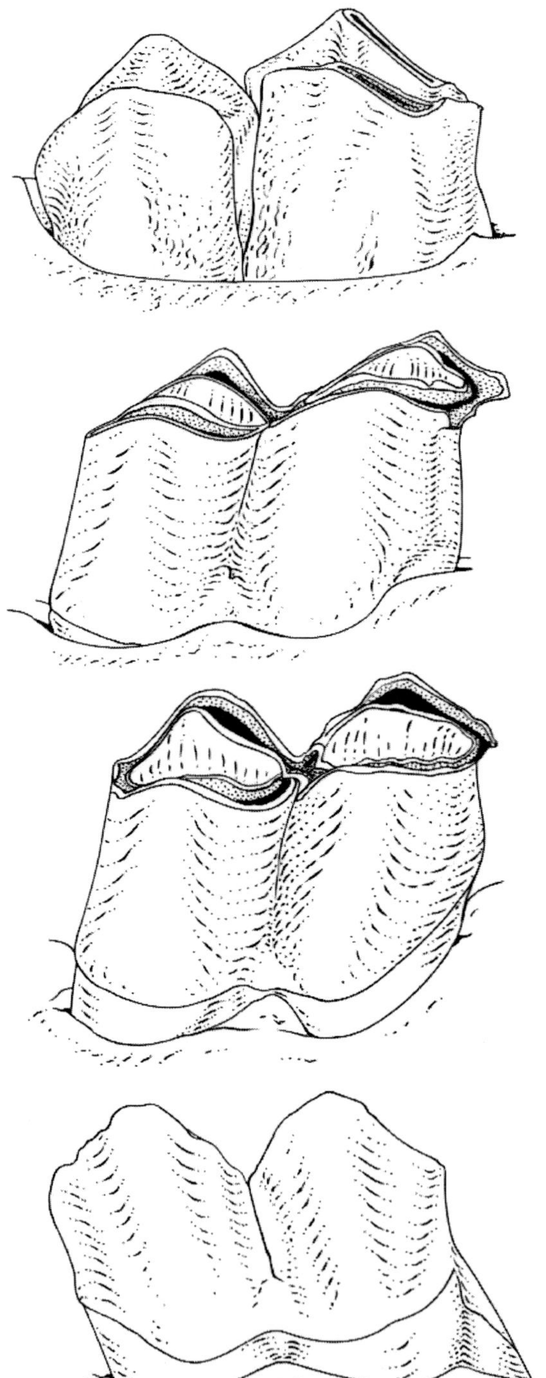

Illustration 7
Roots visible above bone of the alveolar crest

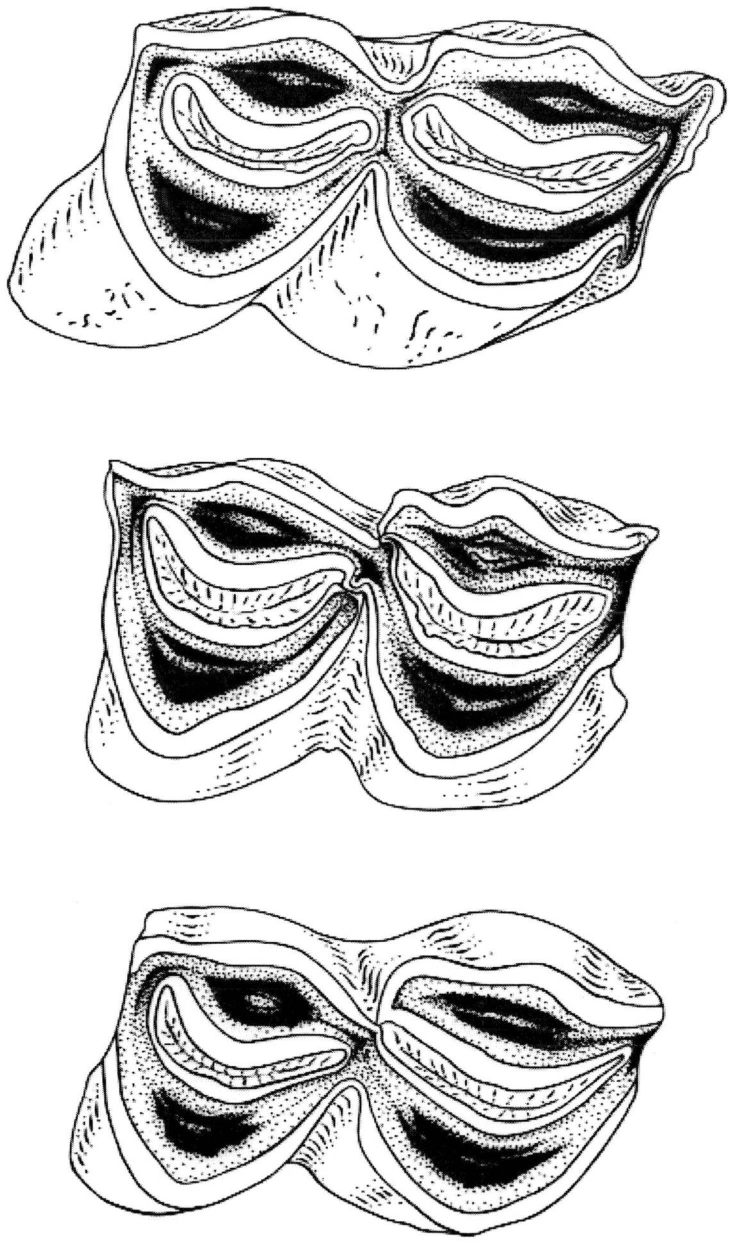

Illustration 8
Enamel lost at contact points between teeth

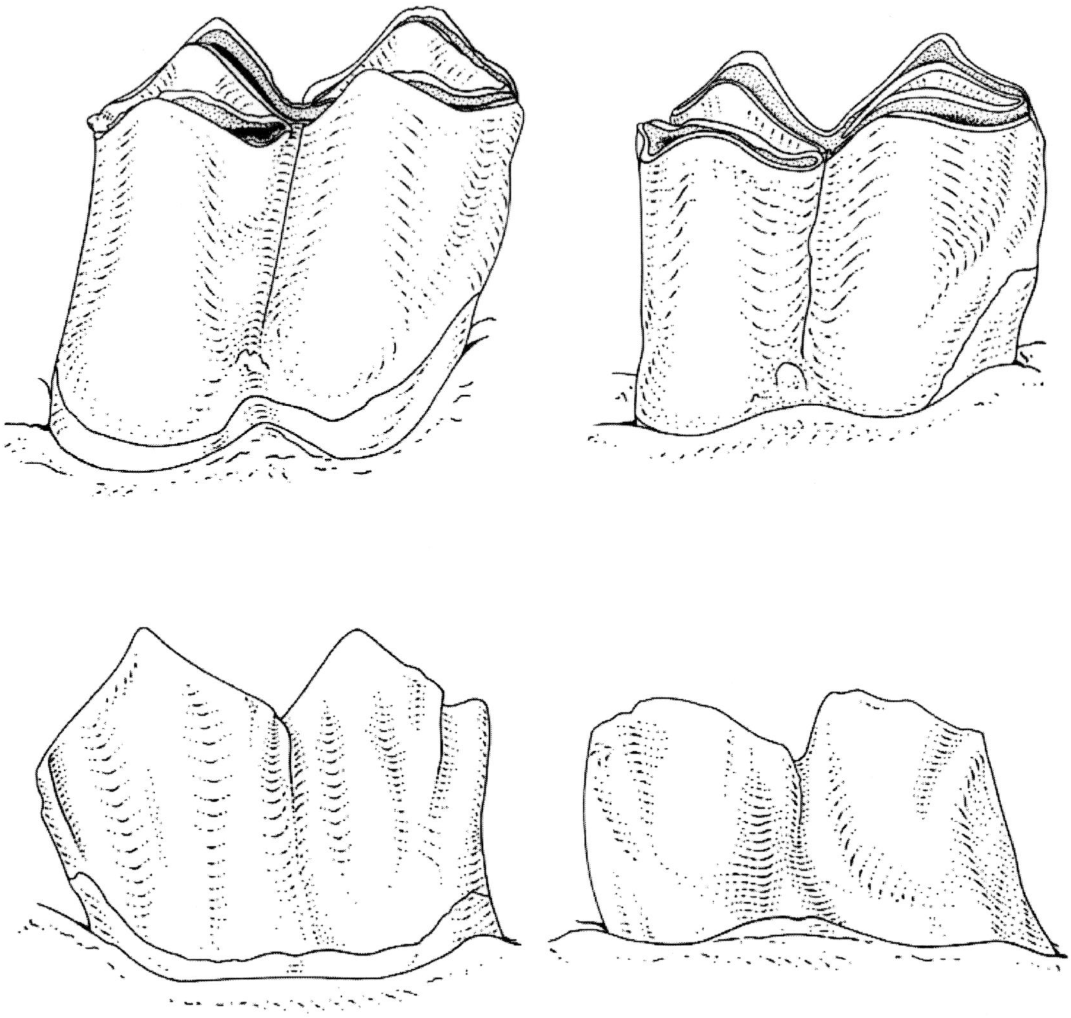

Illustration 9
Acute angle of cusp lips worn to an obtuse angle

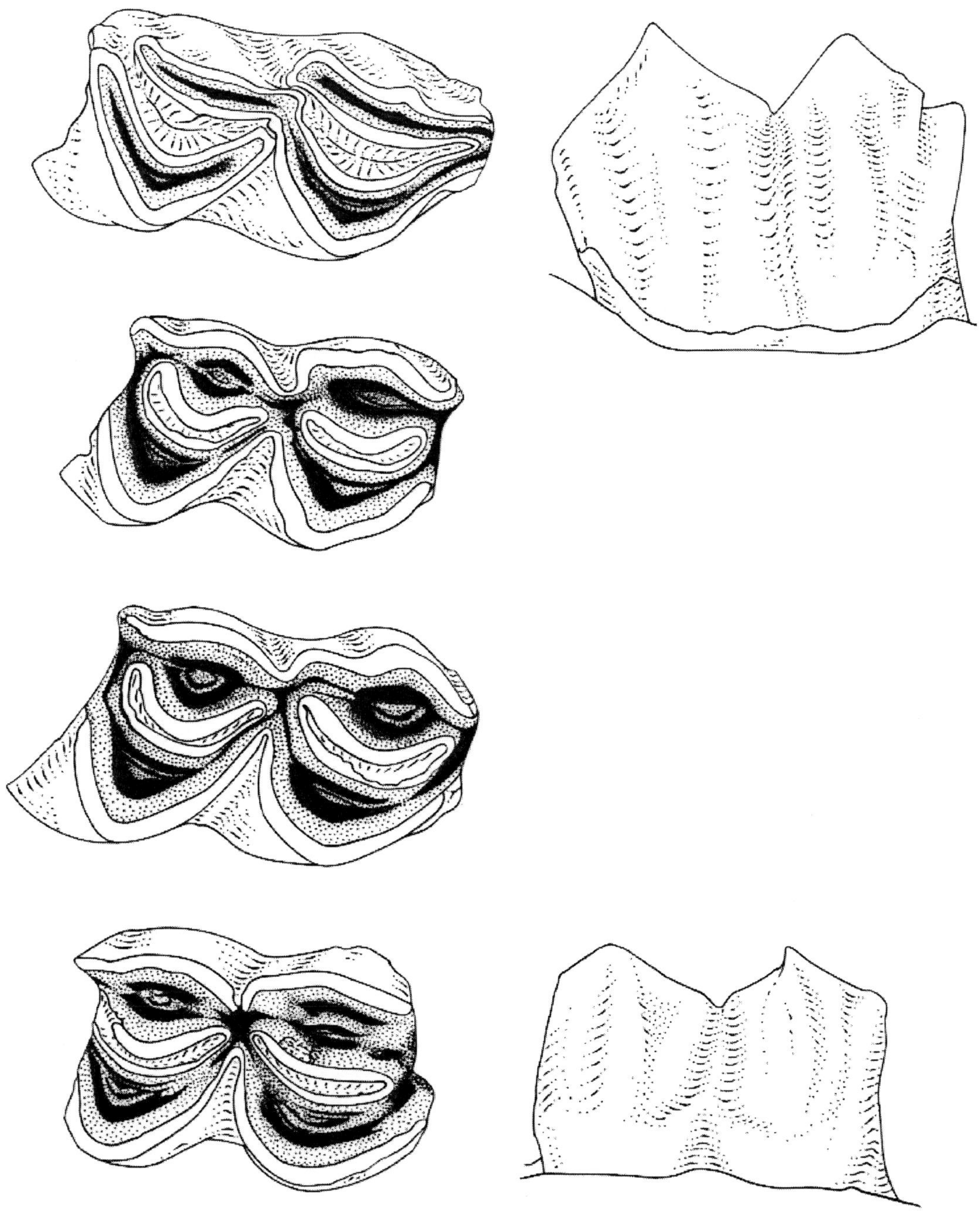

Illustration 10
Loss of vertical lingual crests

Chapter Six
Mathematical basis of the Scoring Scheme

1. INTRODUCTION

In this chapter an alternative method of age estimation, based on tooth wear, is developed. This method takes as its starting point the scoring scheme developed by Brown and Chapman (1991), in which 'scores' are associated to various wear features on the three molars of a jaw being studied. The total score of the jaw, obtained by adding together the scores for those wear features which are present, is correlated with the age of the animal.

The Brown-Chapman scheme provides a reasonably accurate method of ageing, but is nevertheless subject to certain shortcomings which will be addressed in the revised scheme presented here. First, the association of scores to wear features is done on a rather ad hoc basis, with no attempt to ensure that the scores chosen optimize the accuracy of the scheme. Second, the total score obtained does not, in isolation, indicate the age of the animal: in order to obtain an absolute age, it is necessary to associate an age to the score from a graph.

Here, statistical techniques will be used to optimize the weighting associated to the various different scoring elements, in such a way that the final score obtained is an approximation to the age, in months, of the animal under consideration. The aim is to obtain the most accurate scheme possible, subject to the constraint that it be sufficiently simple to be implemented in the field without the benefit of expert training.

The structure of this chapter follows the same four steps that were employed during the research:

1. The first step was to identify the 'scoring elements' that would be used in the scoring scheme: that is, features of a tooth that develop progressively as the animal ages. This was achieved by laying out and studying in detail a large known age sample, covering the whole spectrum from 5 months to over 16 years old. A total of 16 different scoring elements for each molar were identified (with one additional element relating to the hypoconulid of the third molar), only some of which have been used in previous attempts to estimate age from tooth wear. The scoring elements fall into two categories: *discrete* elements, which can take on only whole number values (for example, the number of mesial-distal links, or the number of lingual crests lost), and *continuous* elements, which can take on any value (for example, the crown heights and tooth width). It is clear that discrete elements can in general be measured more rapidly and reliably than continuous ones. These scoring elements are described in detail in chapter 5.

2. Once the scoring elements have been identified, the next step is to work through a known age sample of jaws, determining each of the scoring elements for each of the jaws. These results are recorded on a scoring sheet, as presented in Appendix 3, and transferred to a spreadsheet program. In this case the sample used consisted of the jaws of 41 Highland Red deer of known age, which were kindly provided by the Deer Commission for Scotland.

3. Using this information, a mathematical analysis can be carried out to determine how best to associate *weights* to each of the scoring elements. These determine how significant each element is in obtaining the overall age estimate. For example, if the number of lingual crests lost has weight 2, then a total score of 2 is assigned to each lingual crest lost on each of the three molars. In devising this scheme, a number of criteria were sought in order to ensure that the scheme be simple enough to carry out in the field: a) the weight for each scoring element should be a whole number (if possible, not too large); b) the weights should be independent of the particular molar being studied - thus, for example, there should not be different weights for the number of lingual crests lost on M1 and on M3; c) if possible, the scheme should rely on discrete scoring elements rather than on continuous elements.

4. It is absolutely essential that the scheme be tested on a known age sample other than the one that has been used to choose the weights. Provided that there are enough scoring elements compared to the number of jaws in the sample, weights can always be devised in such a way as to provide a very good correlation between the estimated and actual ages for this particular sample which was used to devise the scheme. The scheme can only be shown to be accurate by testing it on a second, and unrelated, sample. This verification was carried out on a sample of 118 jaws of known age from the Island of Rum, which were made available by the kind permission of Professor Clutton-Brock and Fiona Guinness. I am very grateful to Dr. Barry Brown, who travelled to Rum and scored these jaws on my behalf.

2. DERIVATION OF THE SCORING SCHEME

The sample used to devise the scoring scheme consisted of the jaws of 41 Highland Red deer of known age, which were kindly provided by the Deer Commission for Scotland. A scoring sheet, as presented in Appendix 3, was completed for each of these jaws, and the results entered into a spreadsheet program.

The technique used for deriving the scoring scheme from this data is necessarily mathematical, and is presented formally below for the sake of preciseness. Every effort has been made to make the method accessible to a general reader: additional clarification can be obtained from Appendix 4, in which the steps followed to determine the appropriate weights for each scoring element are described non-mathematically and in detail. For reasons of space and clarity, the data presented in the Appendix is fictitious, and simpler than the actual data obtained from the known aged sample.

It was decided from the outset that the scheme would be devised in such a way that the total score is an approximation to the real age, in months, of the animal. This avoids the need to translate the score to an age, which is not only tedious but also introduces an additional source of potential error. It would have been inappropriate to use years, rather than months, as the unit of measurement: if the weights are to be whole numbers, and the final score were to approximate the age in years of the animal (and so be restricted to a maximum of about 16), then it is clear that almost all of the weights would have to be zero, thus preventing the full range of wear features from being taken into consideration.

Recall that there are 16 distinct scoring elements for each molar, and an additional 17th scoring element for M3, namely the presence or absence of the hypoconulid infundibulum. For the purposes of the statistical development, these scoring elements will be referred to as "scoring element 1", "scoring element 2", and so on up to "scoring element 17". For a given jaw, let $s_{i,j}$ denote the score obtained for scoring element i on molar j, where i lies between 1 and 17, and j between 1 and 3. Thus, for example, $s_{7,2}$ denotes the score obtained on scoring element 7 (the number of infundibula lost) on M2.

As explained in the introduction, it is imposed for the sake of simplicity that the weight associated to each scoring element should be a whole number, and should not depend on the particular molar being scored: thus the weights are given by whole numbers c_i, each bigger than or equal to zero, where i again lies between 1 and 17. Thus, for example, c_7 denotes the weight assigned to scoring element number 7, the number of infundibula lost. These weights have still to be determined: the aim of the statistical analysis is to choose them in such a way as to make the scores obtained for the jaws in the known aged sample approximate their true ages as closely as possible.

An additional constant C is also included, which is again required to be a whole number: this constant gives more flexibility to the scheme, and thus allows a wider possible choice of the weights c_i. The total score assigned to the jaw is then given by

$$S = C + (\sum_{i=1}^{16} c_i(s_{i,1} + s_{i,2} + s_{i,3})) + c_{17}s_{17,3}:$$

that is, the total score S of a given jaw is obtained by scoring each of the sixteen scoring elements on each of the three molars, and the additional seventeenth scoring element for M3, multiplying each of these scores by the appropriate weight for the scoring element, adding all the results, and finally adding the constant C. An example of how this is carried out in practice is given on the simplified scoring sheet at the end of this chapter.

The aim, therefore, is to choose the weights c_i and the constant C in such a way as to minimize the discrepancy between the total scores and the known ages in months, taken over the sample as a whole. In fact, since a sample such as this usually contains erroneous 'outlying' data (perhaps jaws whose known age is incorrectly recorded, which have been incorrectly scored, or which have been subject to some biological condition which renders their tooth wear atypical), the minimization is performed in such a way as to ignore the four worst approximations.

To make the method described above more precise, suppose that for a given choice of weights, the total score of jaw number k in the known age sample is S_k, and that its true age in months is given by T_k (here the number k ranges between 1 and 41, the total number of jaws in the sample). For example, S_{15} and T_{15} denote respectively the total score and the true age in months of the 15th jaw in the sample. The error E_k in the estimation of the age of jaw number k is therefore the difference between S_k and T_k, that is, $E_k = |S_k - T_k|$. Here the vertical lines denote absolute value: the error is always greater than or equal to zero, regardless of which of S_k and T_k is actually larger. Thus, for example, if the 15th jaw in the sample has age 75 months, and the score assigned to it is 70, then E_{15} is equal to 5.

The total error, taken over the whole sample of 41 jaws, is therefore obtained by adding together the individual errors $E_1, E_2, \ldots, E_{41}$. However, as has already been described, it was decided to compensate for possible errors in scoring or in the records of the ages of the jaws, and for animals which for biological reasons have undergone unusual wear, by ignoring the four largest errors in the sample when performing the analysis. The error is therefore given by

$$E = (\sum_{k=1}^{41} E_k) - O,$$

where O, the contribution due to outlyers, is obtained by adding together the four largest values of E_k. In other words, the total error is obtained by adding together the individual errors on 37 of the jaws, ignoring those 4 for which the errors are greatest.

The weights c_i and the constant C have thus to be chosen in such a way as to minimize the total error E: this was performed using the *Solver* feature of the spreadsheet (Microsoft Excel). A detailed description of this process is given in Appendix 4. Because of the size of the sample and the large number (18) of parameters, this calculation takes several hours to perform. However, the results were very satisfactory, yielding a scheme which is simpler than might be expected in the following respects: a) several of the scoring elements were assigned zero weight, and can therefore be ignored in the scheme; b) these ignored scoring elements include all of the continuous elements; and c) the weights assigned, and the constant, are all small numbers (none larger than 3).

The weights assigned were as follows:

Scoring element	*Weight*
Constant	3
Enamel worn	0
Dentine exposed	1
Lingual-buccal links	1
Mesial-distal links	3
Infundibulum closing	3
Infundibulum narrowing****	2
Infundibula lost	0
Hypoconulid infundibulum lost	0
Enamel above bone	0
Contact enamel lost	2
Lingual acute angle lost	2
Buccal acute angle lost	0
Lingual crests lost	2
Dentine width	0
Tooth width	0
Lingual crown height	0
Buccal crown height	0

Table 8: Weights assigned to scoring elements.

A revised scoring sheet can therefore be drawn up, which includes only those scoring elements which feature in the final scheme, and which includes the weights associated to each element. The resulting sheet is included at the end of this chapter, filled in for a sample jaw, with the resulting score recorded.

The following graph shows the true age of each jaw in the sample plotted against its estimated age as obtained using this scoring scheme. As explained in the introduction, it is unsurprising that there is such a good correlation, since the scheme was drawn up precisely in order to ensure strong correlation in this particular sample. The true test of the scheme is when it is applied to a second and unrelated sample: this is carried out in the next section.

Verification of the scheme

As explained in the introduction, the good correlation between true age and estimated age on the sample used to derive the scheme is unsurprising, since the weights have been chosen precisely to obtain a good correlation on this particular sample. In order to verify the accuracy of the scheme, it is absolutely essential that it be tested on a second, and unrelated, sample of known age.

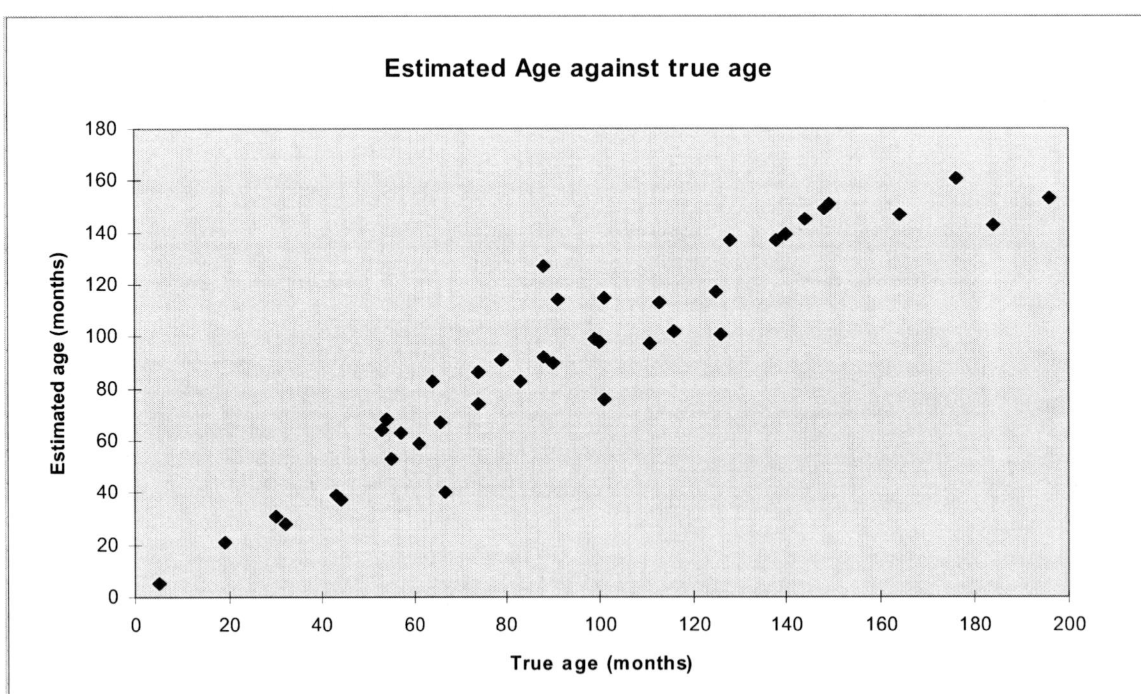

Figure 67: Estimated age using the scoring scheme against the known age.

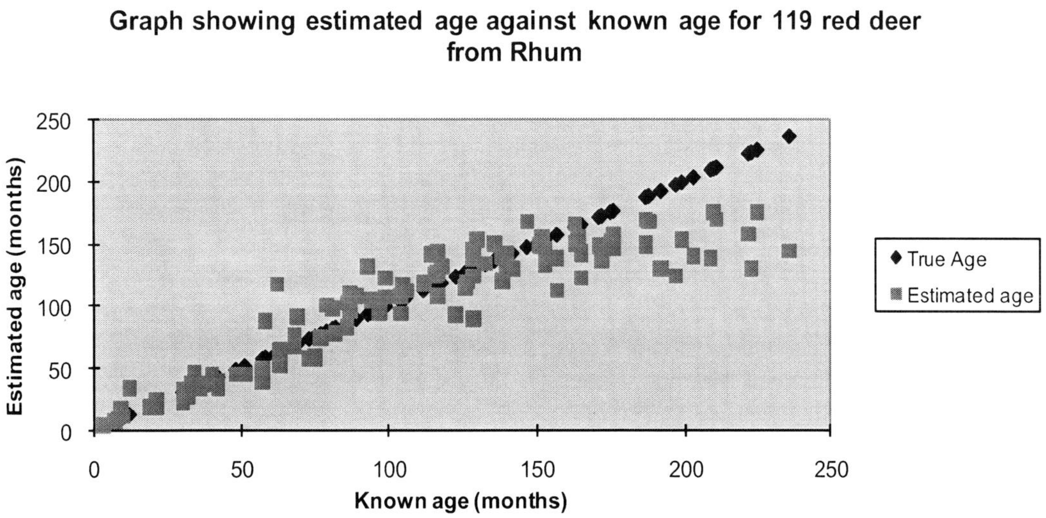

Figure 68: Estimated age using the scoring scheme against known age for 119 Red deer from Rum

This sample consisted of 118 Red deer jaws of known age (between 3 and 236 months) from the Island of Rum, which were made available by the kind permission of Professor Clutton-Brock and Fiona Guinness. The jaws were taken from 65 Female and 53 Male animals, with the majority of the older animals being female. These jaws were scored by Dr. Barry Brown in accordance with the scheme described above, and the scores were then compared with the known ages of the animals. In Chapter 7, it is shown that the interexaminer reliability between Dr. Brown and the author is very good: that is, the two examiners can reliably replicate the same score as each other on a given jaw. The graph above summarizes the results.

The average discrepancy between actual age and estimated age is 17.21 months, and the standard deviation is 18.90 months. It can be seen that the greatest discrepancies occur for the older animals, whose ages are consistently underestimated. The explanation for this is straightforward: by the time an animal reaches about 15 years, its teeth are fully worn, and hence no scheme relying solely on tooth wear can expect to distinguish between animals above this age. If only those 103 animals in the sample which were younger than 15 years are considered, the mean error is reduced to 12.10 months, with a standard deviation of 11.30 months. It is moreover clear from the graph that the great majority of animals under 15 years were aged very accurately (to within 3 or 4 months), and that the relatively large mean error is caused by a much smaller number of animals, whose age estimates were very inaccurate. These could perhaps be accounted for by observer unreliability (see chapter 7), or by atypical wear in the animals themselves. It is certainly possible that the teeth of an individual 5 year old animal can be more worn in every respect than those of typical 7 year old animals, and clearly no ageing technique based on tooth wear would age such an individual accurately.

It is instructive to compare the graph above with the one given below, which shows the buccal and lingual crown heights of the third molar plotted against known age for the same sample of animals. Although crown height is used by many researchers as a means of estimating age, it can be seen readily from the graph that the correlation is in fact very poor.

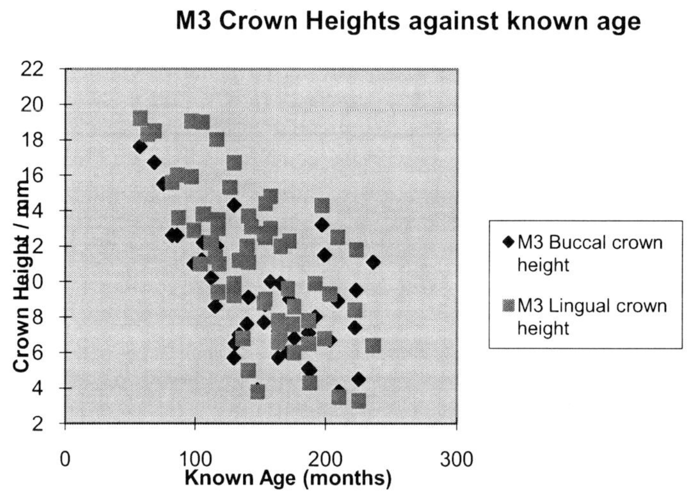

Figure 69: M3 Crown heights against known age

3. CALIBRATION

It must be emphasized that the rate of wear experienced is dependent upon a number of factors, the most obvious being the quality of diet and hardness of food in the environment. It should not therefore be expected that this scoring scheme will provide an accurate absolute assessment of age of animals from environments other than that for which it was developed. It should, however, provide a reasonably accurate relative assessment of age: that is, if one animal has a substantially higher score than a second, one can be confident that it is indeed older.

In making use of this scoring scheme for a given population of Red deer, therefore, it is advisable to begin by calibrating the scheme using as large as possible a sample of known age animals. Ideally, this would be achieved by repeating the analysis employed in this chapter on the given sample, so as to derive a different collection of weights suitable for the environment in question. If this is not practicable, then the weights derived above should be used to score each of the known age jaws, after which jaws of unknown age can be aged approximately by comparing their scores with those of the known age sample.

4. CONCLUSIONS

In this chapter, a new scoring scheme has been described, which both employs more scoring elements, and is derived using more systematic statistical techniques, than previous schemes. Its accuracy, assessed using a sample of known age jaws, has been shown to be better than that of cementum incremental analysis, and it will also be shown in chapter 7 that the scoring scheme is a very much more reliable technique. In addition, it has the advantage that it fast, and does not require expensive equipment or extensive training to implement.

The scores obtained using the scheme are accurate approximations to the age, in months, of highland Red deer. If the animals being aged are from a different environment, then the scheme should be calibrated as described above in order to account for different rates of tooth wear.

SCORING SHEET – HIGHLAND RED DEER

Date: 3/3/98

Scorer: T. D.

Deer identification code: AR 47G

Tag age: 116 months   Date of birth: Date of death:

Sex: Male

Mandible: Right, lower

Provenance: Balmoral

Scoring Element	Range M1/2	Range M3	M1	M2	M3	Total	Weight
Dentine Exposed	0 - 8	0 - 8	4	4	4	12	x 1 = 12
Lingual-Buccal links	0 - 4	0 - 6	4	4	6	14	x 1 = 14
Mesial-Distal links	0 - 2	0 - 6	2	2	6	10	x 3 = 30
Infundibulum closing	0 - 4	0 - 4	4	4	4	12	x 3 = 36
Infundibulum narrowing	0 - 6	0 - 6	2	2	2	6	x 2 = 12
Contact Enamel lost	0 - 2	0 - 1	2	1	0	3	x 2 = 6
Lingual acute angles lost	0 - 2	0 - 2	2	0	0	2	x 2 = 4
Lingual crests lost	0 - 3	0 - 3	1	0	0	1	x 2 = 2
							3
Estimated age in months							119

Figure 70: Revised scoring sheet for highland Red deer

Chapter Seven
Reliability of the Scoring Scheme

1. INTRODUCTION

In the previous chapter, the scoring scheme was shown to give a accurate indication of the relative ages of a collection of animals from a given environment, and of their absolute ages once calibrated against a known age sample from that environment. In this chapter, two aspects of the *reliability* of the scoring scheme are assessed. The first is *intraexaminer reliability*: if a single examiner scores a given jaw independently on several occasions, how reliably will he replicate the same score on each occasion? The second is *interexaminer reliability*: if two trained examiners score the same jaw independently, how reliably will they obtain the same score? It is clear that strong reliability is necessary in both of these scenarios in order for the scoring scheme to be a useful tool in practice.

The measure of reliability which will be employed here is the *intraclass correlation coefficient of reliability (ICC)* (Fleiss 1986), a value between 0 and 1 which gives an indication of how large the variance of the data due to examiner error or uncertainty is as a proportion of the total variance of the data over a large sample of jaws. An ICC close to 1 indicates that the variance due to examiner error is small compared to the total variance, and that reliability is therefore good. The ICC will be discussed briefly in the following section: a good detailed treatment can be found in Fleiss's book (Fleiss 1986), which has been used as the principal source here. I am very grateful to Dr. David Downham and Dr. Toby Hall of the Department of Mathematical Sciences of the University of Liverpool for their help in this respect. Dr. Downham gave invaluable advice on the selection of this relatively unknown statistical technique, and described it to me: a recent paper of his gives an accessible step by step account of this method (Holmbäck, Porter, Downham & Lexell 1999). Dr. Hall helped with the implementation of the method on the data in question.

Once the theoretical background has been established, the reliability of the scoring scheme will be assessed by analyzing a sample of 53 jaws, each of which was independently scored twice by two different examiners. It will be shown that both intraexaminer and interexaminer reliability are very good. These findings are in stark contrast with the similar treatment of cementum incremental analysis given in Chapter 4.

It should be emphasized that reliability is a totally distinct issue from the *accuracy* of the method: for example, an ageing technique which simply declares that every animal is 60 months old is entirely reliable (since every examiner will get the same result on every occasion), but is clearly inaccurate. In order to be useful in practice, a technique must be both accurate and reliable. In fact, the jaws used in the analysis of reliability are of unknown age, so an assessment of accuracy is not possible, even were it desirable.

2. THE INTRACLASS CORRELATION COEFFICIENT (ICC)

Imagine that a single jaw is repeatedly scored under conditions which are as uniform as possible, thus providing a large number of estimates of the age of the animal. The average T of these hypothetical replicate estimates can be regarded as the "true score" of the jaw. An individual score X can differ from T for a number of reasons. The examiner could make a simple error: for example, scoring a feature on the wrong tooth in a jaw, recording the score wrongly on the score sheet, or transcribing it wrongly from the score sheet to a computer for the final analysis. Alternatively, the measurement may have some subjective component: counting the number of acute angles or lingual crests lost on a tooth are good examples of measurements for which there is no well defined dividing line between the feature being present and being absent. Finally, there is an inherent error involved whenever the quantity being measured is continuous (for example, the crown height) rather than discrete (for example, the number of lingual-buccal links). Let e denote the *random error:* that is, the difference, due to all of these combined error effects, between the single observation X and the true score T. Thus X=T+e.

Now consider a large sample of jaws. The true scores T of the different jaws in the sample will vary about some mean value μ with a variance of σ_T^2. For each given jaw, the random error e varies about a mean of zero: under the assumption that the distribution of errors is independent of the true score, the error has a variance of σ_e^2 regardless of the value of T, and hence the total variance of X is

$$\sigma_X^2 = \sigma_T^2 + \sigma_e^2 .$$

That is, there are two components to the variability among a series of measurements on different jaws: variability among their true scores, plus variability of random errors. The relative magnitude of these two effects is expressed by the *Intraclass correlation coefficient of reliability,*

$$R = \frac{\sigma_T^2}{\sigma_T^2 + \sigma_e^2} .$$

Thus the reliability is the proportion of the variance of an observation due to the variation in true scores between different jaws. If the reliability is close to 1, then the error is a small component of the overall variation observed. As is becomes smaller, the error is a larger and larger component of the overall variation: for example, when R=0.5, the variation due to error balances the variation in true scores.

Clearly, there is no well defined criterion for deciding what level of reliability is acceptable: this depends on the particular phenomenon being observed, and the use which will be made of the results. Fleiss (1986, page 7) states that "In general, values of R below 0.4 or so may be taken to represent poor reliability, values above 0.75 or so may be taken to represent excellent reliability, and values between 0.4 and 0.75 may be taken to represent fair to good reliability".

Of more value than a simple reliable/not reliable assessment are that a) the relative reliabilities of two different techniques can be established; and b) if the reliability is known, then it is possible to determine, for example, how many distinct measurements are necessary in order that their average is within a certain tolerance of the true score (see later).

The next issue is to consider how the reliability of the scoring scheme can be calculated. The techniques involved in such a reliability study are most easily understood by means of an example, and the reader is advised to compare the abstract formulation which follows with the specific calculations in the next but one section of this chapter, and with the tutorial treatment which can be found in Appendix 5.

Suppose, then, that each a sample of N jaws is scored k times by a given examiner, with the k different assessments of each jaw carried out, in so far as is possible, independently and under the same conditions. The problem is to estimate the variances σ_T^2 and σ_e^2 of the *population* of jaws from the statistics of the given *sample*.

Consider first of all the total variation between all of the Nk measurements. Let X_{ij} denote the jth measurement on the ith jaw: thus i is a number between 1 and N, and j is a number between 1 and k. The average $\overline{X}$ of these measurements is obtained by adding them all up and dividing by Nk: that is,

$$\overline{X} = \frac{1}{Nk}\sum_{i,j} X_{ij},$$

and an estimate S^2 of the total variance of the population is obtained by adding together the squares of the differences between each measurement and the overall average, and dividing by Nk-1:

$$S^2 = \frac{1}{Nk-1}\sum_{i,j}(X_{ij} - \overline{X})^2.$$

Next, consider the variation due to the different measurements on a given jaw. Let $\overline{X_i}$ be the average of the k distinct scores on the ith jaw: this is the best available estimate of its true score:

$$\overline{X_i} = \frac{1}{k}\sum_{j=1}^{k} X_{ij}.$$

The variance of the distinct measurements on the ith jaw is therefore estimated by

$$s_i^2 = \frac{1}{k-1}\sum_{j=1}^{k}(X_{ij} - \overline{X_i})^2.$$

The best possible estimate of the variation σ_e^2 due to random error, the *within subject mean square* or *WMS*, is obtained by averaging these variances over the jaws in the sample:

$$WMS = \frac{1}{N}\sum_{i=1}^{N} s_i^2.$$

Finally, consider the variation between different jaws in the sample: the *between subjects mean square* or *BMS*, is given by

$$BMS = \frac{k}{N-1}\sum_{i=1}^{N}(\overline{X_i} - \overline{X})^2,$$

and is an estimator for $\sigma_e^2 + k\sigma_T^2$. Notice that this variation necessarily includes a component due to random error: the proportion due to random error decreases as the number k of measurements on each jaw increases. In order to obtain an estimator of the variation σ_T^2 in true scores, we can subtract the WMS from the BMS to obtain an estimator of $k\sigma_T^2$, and then divide by k.

In summary, $s_e^2 = WMS$ is an estimator of σ_e^2, and $s_T^2 = \dfrac{BMS - WMS}{k}$ is an estimator of σ_T^2. Hence an estimator of the reliability R is given by

$$\hat{R} = \frac{s_T^2}{s_T^2 + s_e^2} = \frac{\dfrac{BMS - WMS}{k}}{\dfrac{BMS - WMS}{k} + WMS} = \frac{BMS - WMS}{BMS + (k-1)WMS}$$

It is clear that as the sample size N and the number of measurements k on each jaw become larger, this estimate $\hat{R}$ becomes closer and closer to the true value of the reliability R. In fact (Fleiss 1986 page 12), it is possible to obtain confidence limits for R under the additional assumption that the true score T and the random error e are normally distributed: in this case, a one-sided confidence interval for R at a given level of significance is given by

$$R \geq \frac{\dfrac{BMS}{WMS} - F_{N-1,N(k-1),\alpha}}{\dfrac{BMS}{WMS} + (k-1)F_{N-1,N(k-1),\alpha}},$$

where $F_{N-1,N(k-1),\alpha}$ is the value of the F distribution with N-1 and N(k-1) degrees of freedom which cuts off the proportion α in the upper tail: this can be read off from statistical tables. For example, a 99% confidence interval for R is given by

$$R \geq \frac{\dfrac{BMS}{WMS} - F_{N-1,N(k-1),0.01}}{\dfrac{BMS}{WMS} + (k-1)F_{N-1,N(k-1),0.01}}.$$

The true reliability is at least this great with 99% certainty.

3. INTEREXAMINER RELIABILITY

In the previous section, it was explained how the intraexaminer reliability of the scoring scheme can be assessed. The aim of this section is to extend this treatment to the assessment of interexaminer reliability: that is, to the extent to which two different trained examiners can replicate the same scores on a given sample of jaws. The importance of this assessment, from the point of view of this thesis, is that the known aged jaws used to calibrate the scoring scheme were in fact scored by two different examiners. The scheme would therefore be flawed were the two examiners not scoring consistently with each other.

In order to keep the notation as simple as possible, the theoretical treatment presented here will be restricted to the case (as satisfied by the actual data) in which each of two examiners score each of N jaws independently. Let the true score of the ith jaw be T_i, and suppose that the scores assigned to it by the two examiners are X_i and Y_i. The model which will be used assumes that $X_i = T_i + \lambda + e_i$ and $Y_i = T_i - \lambda + f_i$, where λ is a constant value which expresses the possible different bias of the two examiners, and the random errors e_i and f_i are assumed to be normally distributed with a mean of zero and a variance of σ_e^2 (as in the previous section). There are two important questions to be answered here. First, is there evidence that the two examiners have a significantly different scoring technique: that is, that λ is non-zero? Second, what is the reliability of a set of measurements by the two examiners on a collection of jaws, in which each jaw is studied by only one of the two examiners?

In this case, there are three different causes of variation in the sample data: variation between jaws, variations between examiners, and variations due to random error. Consider first the total variation of the sample: let $\overline{X}$ and $\overline{Y}$ be the averages of the scores provided by the two examiners, and $\overline{Z} = (\overline{X} + \overline{Y})/2$ be the average of their combined scores. Then the total variance of the data is estimated by

$$s^2 = \frac{\sum_{i=1}^{N}(X_i - \overline{Z})^2 + \sum_{i=1}^{N}(Y_i - \overline{Z})^2}{2N-1}.$$

Secondly, consider the variation between jaws: the *jaw mean square* or *JMS* is given by

$$JMS = \frac{2}{N-1}\sum_{i=1}^{N}(\overline{Z_i} - \overline{Z})^2,$$

where $\overline{Z_i}$ is the average of the two examiners' scores for the ith jaw. This is an estimator for $\sigma_e^2 + 2\sigma_T^2$.

Thirdly, consider the variation between examiners. The *scorer mean square*, or *SMS*, is given by

$$SMS = N\left[(\overline{X} - \overline{Z})^2 + (\overline{Y} - \overline{Z})^2\right],$$

and is an estimator for $\sigma_e^2 + 2N\lambda^2$.

Finally, the *error mean square*, or *EMS*, can be calculated by dividing the sum of squares not accounted for by variation between jaws or scorers by the remaining degrees of freedom, namely N-1:

$$EMS = \frac{1}{N-1}\left[(2N-1)s^2 - (N-1)JMS - SMS\right].$$

This is an estimator for σ_e^2.

Provided that the variation between examiners is sufficiently small compared to the variation due to errors, there is no evidence to reject the hypothesis that the examiners have the same scoring technique. This can be tested by comparing the ratio of the two values to tables of the F distribution with 1 and N-1 degrees of freedom. For example, if

$$\frac{SMS}{EMS} \leq F_{1,N-1,0.01},$$

then there is no evidence to reject the hypothesis of same scoring technique at a 99% level of significance.

Now consider the second question: the reliability of a set of measurements obtained on a sample of jaws, each of which is scored by just one of the two examiners. The variance of the measurements obtained in such a study is given by

$$\sigma_X^2 = \sigma_T^2 + \lambda^2 + \sigma_e^2$$

(note that the failure to reject the hypothesis that λ=0 cannot be taken as proof that λ is actually zero). The appropriate version of the intraclass correlation coefficient of reliability, namely the ratio of the variance of true scores to the variance of measured scores, is therefore

$$R = \frac{\sigma_T^2}{\sigma_T^2 + \lambda^2 + \sigma_e^2}.$$

Recalling that *JMS*, *SMS*, and *EMS* are estimators for $\sigma_e^2 + 2\sigma_T^2$, $\sigma_e^2 + 2N\lambda^2$, and σ_e^2 respectively, it follows that an estimator for the reliability is

$$\hat{R} = \frac{\frac{JMS - EMS}{2}}{\frac{JMS - EMS}{2} + \frac{SMS - EMS}{2N} + EMS} = \frac{N(JMS - EMS)}{N(JMS - EMS) + (SMS - EMS) + 2N \cdot EMS}$$

$$= \frac{N(JMS - EMS)}{N \cdot JMS + SMS + (N-1)EMS}.$$

4. THE SAMPLE

A sample of 53 jaws was studied by two examiners, the author (examiner 1) and Dr. Barry Brown, a dental anatomist (examiner 2). Each examiner scored each of the jaws twice, with an interval of at least a week between successive scorings of the same jaw. No reference was made to the results of the first score while carrying out the second. The jaws were labelled with long and unmemorable codes, in order to ensure that the examiners would not be able to remember the scores which they had previously assigned them.

The following table records the two age estimates obtained by each of the two examiners. For reasons of space, the detailed breakdown of the different elements of the scoring scheme is not included, although each of these elements will be given an independent reliability analysis in the following section.

	Examiner 1		Examiner 2	
Code	Score 1	Score 2	Score 1	Score 2
5678ABCDEF	93	90	94	92
5ABCDE678F	53	47	42	49
5ABCDEF678	68	64	62	64
5ABCDF678E	11	11	11	12
5ABCFE678D	68	71	61	77
5ABDFE678C	147	147	151	151
5ACDFE678B	60	52	50	54
5BCDFE678A	133	129	133	127
678ABCDEF5	68	67	58	64
6ABCDE578F	138	130	137	144
6ABCDF578E	181	183	183	177
6ABCFE578D	108	111	123	111
6ABDFE578C	39	39	35	38
6ACDFE378B	94	86	94	104
6BCDFE578A	108	100	117	123
78ABCDEF56	80	71	79	89
7ABCDE568F	143	129	141	127
7ABCDEF56D	73	49	40	53
7ABCDF568E	75	69	74	83
8ABCDEF567	115	95	95	93
A5BCDEF678	39	42	42	48
A68CDEF578	79	76	96	91
A7BCDEF568	115	94	101	94
ABCDEFGH	120	114	112	121
B5ACDEF678	133	127	139	135
B6ACDEF578	75	77	86	85
B8ACDEF567	91	87	85	105
BCDEF5678A	126	111	128	129
BCDEFGHA	74	73	62	73
C5ADEF678B	117	108	116	123
C6ADEFB785	80	78	70	76
C785ABDEF6	111	112	130	132
CDEF5678AB	112	115	114	122
CDEFGHAB	68	69	47	57
D756ABDEF8	82	76	82	84
D785ABDEF6	113	98	116	119
D786ABDEF5	87	89	97	93
DEF5678ABC	173	169	171	173
DEFGHABC	141	133	153	147
E678ABCDF5	67	74	72	74
E765ABDEF8	131	112	123	107
E785ABDEF6	90	84	95	90
E786ABDEF5	75	74	60	77
EF5678ABCD	147	129	131	132
EFGHABCD	88	94	98	98
F5678ABCDE	86	81	78	76
F567ABCDE8	52	48	41	50
F678ABDE5	49	50	48	50
F785ABCDE6	11	11	9	11
F8765ABCDE	22	18	18	18
FGHABCDE	139	125	126	121
GHABCDEF	133	121	111	120
HABCDEFG	116	105	110	112

Table 9: Age estimates by two examiners using the scoring scheme

5. INTRAEXAMINER RELIABILITY

To determine the reliability of each of the two examiners, the prescription in the section on the intraclass correlation coefficient should be followed. It is hoped that the application of this method as described in this section will convince the reader who lacks the statistical background to follow the theoretical argument that the reliability is nevertheless relatively straightforward to calculate in practice. A tutorial guide to this technique, presented using simplified data, is given in Appendix 5.

Consider first the reliability of examiner 1. In this case, N=53 (the number of jaws in the sample), and k=2 (the number of times examiner 1 repeated the scoring). The average $\overline{X}$ of all 106 scores is obtained by adding them all up and dividing by 106: for this data, which is displayed again in the second and third columns of the table below, $\overline{X} = 91.61$. The next step is to calculate the values $\overline{X_i}$: that is, the average for each jaw of the two scores obtained for it. Thus, for example, $\overline{X_1}$ is the average of 93 and 90, namely 91.5. These averages are given in the fourth column of the table below. Then the estimator s_i^2 of the variance of distinct scores on the ith jaw is given by taking each of the two scores in turn, subtracting it from the mean score for that jaw, squaring the result, and adding the numbers obtained for the two scores. Since k-1=1, no division is necessary. Thus, for example,

$s_1^2 = (91.5-90)^2 + (91.5-93)^2 = (1.5)^2 + (1.5)^2 = 2.25 + 2.25 = 4.5$

.

Notice that, because there are only two measurements on each jaw, the two squares which are added in this calculation are always the same. The values of s_i^2 are given in the fifth column of the following table. Once these have been calculated, the within subjects mean square can be calculated by adding together these 53 values of s_i^2 and dividing by 53. In this case, the value obtained for WMS is 39.52.

Finally, to calculate the BMS, it is necessary to calculate $\sum_{i=1}^{N}(\overline{X_i} - \overline{X})^2$.

The sixth column in the table below gives the values of $\overline{X_i} - \overline{X}$: for each jaw, the overall average score 91.61 is subtracted from the average of the two scores for that jaw. The final column gives the squares of these values. The BMS is obtained by adding together all the values in this final column, multiplying by k (=2) and dividing by N-1 (=52). In this case, BMS=2775.28

Hence the estimator of the reliability R is given by

$$\hat{R} = \frac{BMS - WMS}{BMS + (2-1)WMS} = \frac{2775.28 - 39.52}{2775.28 + 39.52} \approx 0.9719.$$

Code	Score 1	Score 2	Average	Variance	Av-Ov Av	(Av-Ov Av)^2
5678ABCDEF	93	90	91.5	4.5	91.5	8372.25
5ABCDE678F	53	47	50	18	50	2500
5ABCDEF678	68	64	66	8	66	4356
5ABCDF678E	11	11	11	0	11	121
5ABCFE678D	68	71	69.5	4.5	69.5	4830.25
5ABDFE678C	147	147	147	0	147	21609
5ACDFE678B	60	52	56	32	56	3136
5BCDFE678A	133	129	131	8	131	17161
678ABCDEF5	68	67	67.5	0.5	67.5	4556.25
6ABCDE578F	138	130	134	32	134	17956
6ABCDF578E	181	183	182	2	182	33124
6ABCFE578D	108	111	109.5	4.5	109.5	11990.25
6ABDFE578C	39	39	39	0	39	1521
6ACDFE378B	94	86	90	32	90	8100
6BCDFE578A	108	100	104	32	104	10816
78ABCDEF56	80	71	75.5	40.5	75.5	5700.25
7ABCDE568F	143	129	136	98	136	18496
7ABCDEF56D	73	49	61	288	61	3721
7ABCDF568E	75	69	72	18	72	5184
8ABCDEF567	115	95	105	200	105	11025
A5BCDEF678	39	42	40.5	4.5	40.5	1640.25
A68CDEF578	79	76	77.5	4.5	77.5	6006.25
A7BCDEF568	115	94	104.5	220.5	104.5	10920.25
ABCDEFGH	120	114	117	18	117	13689
B5ACDEF678	133	127	130	18	130	16900
B6ACDEF578	75	77	76	2	76	5776
B8ACDEF567	91	87	89	8	89	7921
BCDEF5678A	126	111	118.5	112.5	118.5	14042.25
BCDEFGHA	74	73	73.5	0.5	73.5	5402.25
C5ADEF678B	117	108	112.5	40.5	112.5	12656.25
C6ADEFB785	80	78	79	2	79	6241
C785ABDEF6	111	112	111.5	0.5	111.5	12432.25
CDEF5678AB	112	115	113.5	4.5	113.5	12882.25
CDEFGHAB	68	69	68.5	0.5	68.5	4692.25
D756ABDEF8	82	76	79	18	79	6241
D785ABDEF6	113	98	105.5	112.5	105.5	11130.25
D786ABDEF5	87	89	88	2	88	7744
DEF5678ABC	173	169	171	8	171	29241
DEFGHABC	141	133	137	32	137	18769

E678ABCDF5	67	74	70.5	24.5	70.5	4970.25
E765ABDEF8	131	112	121.5	180.5	121.5	14762.25
E785ABDEF6	90	84	87	18	87	7569
E786ABDEF5	75	74	74.5	0.5	74.5	5550.25
EF5678ABCD	147	129	138	162	138	19044
EFGHABCD	88	94	91	18	91	8281
F5678ABCDE	86	81	83.5	12.5	83.5	6972.25
F567ABCDE8	52	48	50	8	50	2500
F678ABDE5	49	50	49.5	0.5	49.5	2450.25
F785ABCDE6	11	11	11	0	11	121
F8765ABCDE	22	18	20	8	20	400
FGHABCDE	139	125	132	98	132	17424
GHABCDEF	133	121	127	72	127	16129
HABCDEFG	116	105	110.5	60.5	110.5	12210.25

Table 10: Determination of first examiner's reliability.

These calculations, while extremely laborious to carry out by hand, are made very straightforward by the use of a spreadsheet program.

The value obtained is only an estimate for the true reliability of the first examiner. As explained above, a 99% confidence interval for the true value of R can be calculated by

$$R \geq \frac{\frac{BMS}{WMS} - F_{N-1,N(k-1),0.01}}{\frac{BMS}{WMS} + (k-1)F_{N-1,N(k-1),0.01}}.$$

In this case, N=53 and k=2. The value of $F_{52,53,0.01}$ can be looked up in statistical tables, and is 1.915. Therefore

$$R \geq \frac{\frac{2775.28}{39.52} - 1.915}{\frac{2775.28}{39.52} + 1.915} \approx 0.947$$

with 99% confidence.

Exactly the same calculations can be repeated for the scores obtained by examiner 2, to obtain an estimate of 0.981 for his reliability, and $R \geq 0.964$ with 99% confidence.

6. RELIABILITY OF INDIVIDUAL SCORING ELEMENTS

In the previous section, the reliability of the two examiners' assessments of the total score of a jaw was calculated. Here the same treatment will be applied to each of the individual components measured in the scoring process: the aim is to determine whether or not some aspects of the process are significantly less reliable than others. It will be assumed that reliability in scoring a feature does not depend on the particular tooth in the jaw being scored, and hence only the scores for M1 will be used (with the exception, of course, of the presence or absence of the hypoconulid infundibulum). The method of analysis is exactly the same as in the previous section: the only change is that, instead of using the total scores as the starting data, the scores for a particular scoring element are used instead. The results obtained are given in the following table.

	Examiner 1			Examiner 2		
Element	Reliability	95%	99%	Reliability	95%	99%
Enamel Worn	0.986	0.978	0.973	0.980	0.968	0.961
Dentine Exposed *	1	1	1	1	1	1
Lingual-Buccal links *	0.953	0.927	0.912	0.953	0.927	0.912
Mesial-Distal links *	0.890	0.831	0.799	0.858	0.785	0.745
Infundibula closing *	0.972	0.956	0.947	0.925	0.883	0.860
Infundibula narrowing *	0.771	0.661	0.603	0.921	0.878	0.854
Infundibula lost	1	1	1	0.823	0.733	0.686
Enamel above bone	0.802	0.704	0.652	0.714	0.583	0.516
Contact enamel lost *	0.591	0.422	0.340	0.656	0.506	0.431
Acute angle lingual *	0.623	0.464	0.385	0.871	0.804	0.767
Acute angle buccal	0.544	0.364	0.277	0.548	0.368	0.282
Lingual crests lost *	0.769	0.658	0.600	0.646	0.493	0.417
Hypoconulid infundibulum lost	0.655	0.505	0.430	0.825	0.737	0.690

Table 11: Reliability of individual scoring elements

The scoring elements marked with an asterisk in the above table are those which are actually used in the final computation of the score. It is interesting to note that most of the individual reliabilities of these elements are less than the overall reliability of the scheme. The most likely explanation for this is that errors made in the analysis tend to cancel one another out rather than to accumulate.

7. INTEREXAMINER RELIABILITY

The next step is to consider the interexaminer reliability: to decide whether or not the two examiners are scoring equivalently, and to determine the reliability of the scores on a sample of jaws in which each jaw is scored by only one of the two examiners (effectively chosen at random). The second and third columns of the following table give the scores assigned to each of the 53 jaws by the two examiners (in each case, calculated as the average of their two independent scorings of the jaw). These are the random variables X_i and Y_i: thus, for example, $X_1 = 91.5$ and $Y_1 = 93$. The average of the first examiner's scores is $\overline{X} = 91.61$, and that of the second examiner's scores is $\overline{Y} = 92.66$. The overall average of all 106 scores is thus $\overline{Z} = 92.14$ (the average of 91.61 and 92.66). The total variance is estimated by

$$s^2 = \frac{\sum_{i=1}^{N}(X_i - \overline{Z})^2 + \sum_{i=1}^{N}(Y_i - \overline{Z})^2}{2N-1}.$$

The fourth column of the table gives the values of $\left(X_i - \overline{Z}\right)^2$: they are calculated by subtracting 92.14 from the values in the second column, and squaring the result. Similarly, the values in the fifth column are obtained by subtracting 92.14 from the values in the third column, and squaring the result. The estimate of the total variance is obtained by adding together all 106 values in these two columns, and dividing by 105. This gives $s^2 = 1447.92$.

Consider next the Jaw mean square

$$JMS = \frac{2}{N-1}\sum_{i=1}^{N}(\overline{Z_i} - \overline{Z})^2.$$

The sixth column of the table gives the values of $\overline{Z_i}$, obtained by taking the average of the values in the second and third columns. The seventh column is obtained by subtracting 92.14 from these values, and squaring the result. The Jaw mean square is obtained by adding together all of the values in the seventh column, multiplying by 2 and dividing by 52: this gives a value for JMS of 2892.38.

Next, the scorer mean square is given by

$$SMS = N\left[(\overline{X} - \overline{Z})^2 + (\overline{Y} - \overline{Z})^2\right] = 53\left[(91.61 - 92.14)^2 + (92.66 - 92.14)^2\right] = 3.983,$$

and finally the error mean square is

$$EMS = \frac{1}{N-1}\left[(2N-1)s^2 - (N-1)JMS - SMS\right] = \frac{1}{52}\left[105s^2 - 52JMS - SMS\right] = 31.22.$$

It can be seen that SMS is extremely small compared to EMS (in fact SMS/EMS is about 0.128), and hence there will be no evidence to reject the hypothesis of equal examiner effects even at a very high level of significance. For example, at the 99.9% level of significance this ratio should be compared to $F_{1,52,0.001} = 12.16$.

Finally, an estimate of the reliability of joint measurements by the two examiners is given by

$$\hat{R} = \frac{N(JMS - EMS)}{N \cdot JMS + SMS + (N-1)EMS},$$

which in this case evaluates to 0.979.

Code	Mean 1	Mean 2	Square 1	Square 2	Overall mean	Square
5678ABCDEF	91.5	93	8372.25	8649	92.25	8510.062
5ABCDE678F	50	45.5	2500	2070.25	47.75	2280.062
5ABCDEF678	66	63	4356	3969	64.5	4160.25
5ABCDF678E	11	11.5	121	132.25	11.25	126.5625
5ABCFE678D	69.5	69	4830.25	4761	69.25	4795.562
5ABDFE678C	147	151	21609	22801	149	22201
5ACDFE678B	56	52	3136	2704	54	2916
5BCDFE678A	131	130	17161	16900	130.5	17030.25
678ABCDEF5	67.5	61	4556.25	3721	64.25	4128.062
6ABCDE578F	134	140.5	17956	19740.25	137.25	18837.56

6ABCDE578F	134	140.5	17956	19740.25	137.25	18837.56
6ABCDF578E	182	180	33124	32400	181	32761
6ABCFE578D	109.5	117	11990.25	13689	113.25	12825.56
6ABDFE578C	39	36.5	1521	1332.25	37.75	1425.062
6ACDFE378B	90	99	8100	9801	94.5	8930.25
6BCDFE578A	104	120	10816	14400	112	12544
78ABCDEF56	75.5	84	5700.25	7056	79.75	6360.062
7ABCDE568F	136	134	18496	17956	135	18225
7ABCDEF56D	61	46.5	3721	2162.25	53.75	2889.062
7ABCDF568E	72	78.5	5184	6162.25	75.25	5662.562
8ABCDEF567	105	94	11025	8836	99.5	9900.25
A5BCDEF678	40.5	45	1640.25	2025	42.75	1827.562
A68CDEF578	77.5	93.5	6006.25	8742.25	85.5	7310.25
A7BCDEF568	104.5	97.5	10920.25	9506.25	101	10201
ABCDEFGH	117	116.5	13689	13572.25	116.75	13630.56
B5ACDEF678	130	137	16900	18769	133.5	17822.25
B6ACDEF578	76	85.5	5776	7310.25	80.75	6520.562
B8ACDEF567	89	95	7921	9025	92	8464
BCDEF5678A	118.5	128.5	14042.25	16512.25	123.5	15252.25
BCDEFGHA	73.5	67.5	5402.25	4556.25	70.5	4970.25
C5ADEF678B	112.5	119.5	12656.25	14280.25	116	13456
C6ADEFB785	79	73	6241	5329	76	5776
C785ABDEF6	111.5	131	12432.25	17161	121.25	14701.56
CDEF5678AB	113.5	118	12882.25	13924	115.75	13398.06
CDEFGHAB	68.5	52	4692.25	2704	60.25	3630.062
D756ABDEF8	79	83	6241	6889	81	6561
D785ABDEF6	105.5	117.5	11130.25	13806.25	111.5	12432.25
D786ABDEF5	88	95	7744	9025	91.5	8372.25
DEF5678ABC	171	172	29241	29584	171.5	29412.25
DEFGHABC	137	150	18769	22500	143.5	20592.25
E678ABCDF5	70.5	73	4970.25	5329	71.75	5148.062
E765ABDEF8	121.5	115	14762.25	13225	118.25	13983.06
E785ABDEF6	87	92.5	7569	8556.25	89.75	8055.062
E786ABDEF5	74.5	68.5	5550.25	4692.25	71.5	5112.25
EF5678ABCD	138	131.5	19044	17292.25	134.75	18157.56
EFGHABCD	91	98	8281	9604	94.5	8930.25
F5678ABCDE	83.5	77	6972.25	5929	80.25	6440.062
F567ABCDE8	50	45.5	2500	2070.25	47.75	2280.062
F678ABDE5	49.5	49	2450.25	2401	49.25	2425.562
F785ABCDE6	11	10	121	100	10.5	110.25
F8765ABCDE	20	18	400	324	19	361
FGHABCDE	132	123.5	17424	15252.25	127.75	16320.06
GHABCDEF	127	115.5	16129	13340.25	121.25	14701.56
HABCDEFG	110.5	111	12210.25	12321	110.75	12265.56

Table 12: Determination of interexaminer reliability

8. CONCLUSIONS

In this treatment, it has been shown that both intraexaminer and interexaminer reliability for the scoring scheme are extremely good. This means that the scheme, given that it is also accurate, is useful in practice – a single examiner can reliably obtain the same score when examining the same jaw on two different occasions, and a large sample of jaws can be divided between two or more examiners to be scored, without any significant bias being introduced due to variability between examiners. These finding are in stark contrast to the results of the similar analysis of cementum incremental analysis presented in Chapter 4.

Chapter Eight
Summary and Conclusions

1. OVERVIEW

The principal intention of this research was to study the extent to which cementum incremental analysis can be used to determine the age and season of death of Red deer, using techniques which are applicable to archaeological material. Age and seasonality determination are of great importance in archaeology, providing information about prehistoric hunting strategies, and settlement and subsistence patterns; they are also of current interest to wildlife managers. The results which have been presented, in so far as they pertain to incremental analysis, are largely negative - some of the more important points (discussed in more detail below) are:

- There is no doubt that incremental structures exist in Red deer cementum. However there is no agreement about either the nature or the causes of these structures, and in particular there is no strong evidence for seasonal deposition. (Chapter 1).
- It is clear, since the incremental structure is laid down over time, that there must be some correlation between the number of bands and lines which can be observed and the age of the animal. However the number of layers typically varies substantially between different locations on the tooth, and the studies presented here showed no consistent agreement, at any given location, between the number of layers and the age in years of the animal. There was also no consistent correlation between the outermost layer and the season of death. (Chapter 4, Appendix 6).
- The subjective nature of incremental analysis is shown by reliability studies: a trained examiner cannot reliably replicate his measurements on a given specimen. This situation may be improved by the use of confocal microscopy and computer image enhancement, both of which can improve the definition of the image. (Chapter 4).
- These problems are compounded, particularly when comparing the work of different researchers, by a lack of uniformity in the method of preparation of thin sections, in microscopical technique, and in terminology. (Chapters 1 and 3).

I strongly recommend, on the basis of these findings, that valuable archaeological material should not be subjected to sectioning until a great deal of further research has been carried out on modern samples, preferably with known ages and life histories. Some suggestions for such research are presented at the end of this chapter. Moreover, I do not believe, on the basis of the research presented here, that incremental analysis can ever provide accurate seasonality assessments for archaeological Red deer. However, this is not in any way to suggest that incremental analysis is not a suitable subject of study for archaeologists, still less for wildlife biologists who are not restricted to the use of standard ground thin sections (see Chapter 3). In the first place, it should be stressed that this research is specific to Red deer (although it seems probable that most of the points outlined above will be applicable to other mammals). More importantly, however, it seems likely that the incremental structure does reflect one or more "basic events in an animal's life" (Klevezal 1970). If more detailed experimentation were to reveal what these basic events are, and how they are reflected, then incremental analysis would provide an immensely valuable tool for understanding the life histories of animals in the archaeological context.

The second part of the research presented here describes a new scoring scheme for estimating the age of highland Red deer on the basis of tooth wear. Tooth wear is clearly subject to many 'random' external influences, and hence can never provide a truly accurate means of ageing, still less of seasonality determination. It is shown in this thesis, however, that it is both a more accurate and a more reliable means of ageing than cementum incremental analysis: it also has the benefits of being quick, easy to learn, cheap, and, most importantly, non-destructive. I would recommend that, at least for the time being, this method be used for building up age profiles from archaeological sites.

2. CEMENTUM INCREMENTAL ANALYSIS – A REVIEW

The possibility of being able to determine the age and season of death, or to understand other aspects of the life history of an animal, by study of the incremental structure of its cementum is very exciting, and it is unsurprising that this area of research has attracted the interest of archaeologists: very little evidence is available which permits a thorough understanding of seasonal movement by prehistoric populations. However, there are many problems with cementum incremental analysis, associated, amongst other things, with the nature of cementum (and the causes and complexity of incremental structures in cementum), and the subjectivity of interpretation. In this section, the principal problems that have been described in this thesis are summarised.

Cementum and its incremental structures

Neither cementum itself, the "least-known mineralized tissue" (Bosshardt and Schroeder 1996), nor the incremental structures which it exhibits, are well understood. There are two aspects to the understanding of incremental structures: their nature (the biological structures which give rise to alternating bands and lines) and their causes (the external and internal stimuli which induce layering). Little research has been devoted to the nature of increments: amongst the conjectures which have been made are that the different optical properties of bands and lines are due to differences in calcium content (McLaren 1958, Sergeant 1959, 1962, Berzin 1961, 1964, Kubota et al 1963, Ohsumi et al 1963, Klevezal and Kleinberg 1967); to differences in density due to different mineralization rates, associated to different proportions of extrinsic and intrinsic fibres (Klevezal and Kleinberg 1967, Boyde and Jones 1972, Jones 1981, Davis 1986, Hillson 1986); and to differences in orientation of the Sharpey's fibres (Lieberman 1993, 1994). Similarly, a large number of conjectures have been put forward for the causes of incremental structures (nutrition, biomechanical changes, hormonal changes, climatic changes, and metabolic changes), but few experiments have been carried out to determine which one or more of these factors is decisive (see however Lieberman 1993).

Of course, the lack of understanding of the nature and causes of increments would not hinder the *application* of cementum incremental analysis were it possible to associate the transitions between bands and lines to well-defined life events, such as the changing seasons or the rut (notice that such life events typically impact upon several of the proposed causes listed above). Unfortunately, however, although many researchers work on the assumption that incremental structures are seasonal, no such correlation with life events has been established. The difficulty of making such a correlation in general is made clear by the lack of uniformity of cementum distribution around the tooth root: many authors have observed that the number of bands and lines, and their widths, can vary substantially at different locations around the root, as well as between different teeth of the same animal. This problem is discussed in detail in Chapter 4, where sections from a known-aged sample are considered individually and in detail. The discrepancy in the incremental structure around the root is also highlighted by the data from a larger sample of 120 sections, which is presented in Appendix 6. Each section in the sample was studied at each of 11 different standard locations, and it was found (see Table 17) that the average discrepancy between the smallest and the largest number of bands observed at different locations is 3.25. On average, therefore, if a section is examined carefully around the whole of the tooth root, there will be an ambiguity of more than three years in the resulting age estimate. Moreover, the discrepancy between the smallest and largest number of bands observed was more than 5 bands in over 15% of the sample.

The difficulty of interpretation of the incremental structure is compounded by the existence of false, split, and secondary increments whose causes are equally poorly understood, and which require some experience (and a complete tooth) to identify; and by the phenomenon of cementum resorption. In the archaeological context, it is also necessary to consider taphonomic factors: little systematic research has been carried out on how prolonged exposure of jaws or isolated teeth affects the incremental structure of cementum.

Problems of Interpretation

The unevenness of cementum distribution (and in particular of the number of observed bands and lines) around a tooth root has already been mentioned, and is clearly the greatest single obstacle to interpreting the incremental structure of a given tooth. A number of authors have commented on the necessity of studying the whole root, but those who attempt to make age assessments generally either default to the area of 'best fit' (without stating what it fits best with - presumably the known age of the animal), or to the area where the incremental structure is clearest (although there is no reason why this should give a more accurate age assessment than any other location). As is explained in Chapter 4 and in Appendix 6, there does not appear to be any one location on the root that consistently exhibits a number of bands and lines which corresponds to the age of the animal. It is also argued in Appendix 6 that there is no location at which the age of the animal is well correlated with the number of bands and lines, even allowing for relationships which are more complicated than that which arises from one band and one line being laid down each year.

Another problem arises from the subjective nature of observation of incremental structures: a reliability study of age estimation by incremental analysis is presented. It is shown that, using an optical microscope with polarised transmitted light, the reliability of age estimation is less than 50%. This statement has nothing to do with the accuracy of the method: it concerns the inability of a trained examiner to replicate his age assessments when studying the same section on two different occasions. The interpretation of the statement is that, when analysing a large sample of teeth, the variability of measurements due to examiner unreliability is greater than the variability due to differences between the different teeth in the sample. The reliability can doubtless be improved: it was found that the use of confocal microscopy and computer image enhancement can both improve the definition of the image. However it should be stressed that this only makes the identification of bands and lines more objective: it does not help to understand what they represent, or to remove the disparity between what is seen at different locations around the root.

Other Issues

Three other issues have been stressed throughout this thesis. First, it is clearly important, if one wishes to draw conclusions about the life history of an unknown animal by incremental analysis, to have studied a large sample of animals of the same species which are of known age (preferably tagged at birth) and, if possible, known life history. Such samples are rare and valuable, and it can be difficult to persuade their guardians to give them up for research which involves their destruction. Second, the confusion surrounding the identification and interpretation of incremental structures is exacerbated by inconsistent terminology (sometimes bewilderingly complicated), and different techniques of section preparation and examination (which are frequently undocumented). Third, accurate incremental analysis, which involves careful section preparation and an informed understanding of what is being seen through the microscope, cannot be carried out without thorough training.

3. THE SCORING SCHEME

In Chapters 5 and 6 a new scoring scheme for estimating the age of Red deer by means of tooth wear is presented. This scheme takes as its starting point the work of Brown and Chapman (1991). Sixteen *scoring elements* (features of a tooth that develop progressively as the animal ages) were identified, and a statistical analysis was performed in order to assign *weights* to each of the scoring elements, in such a way that the age of an animal in months can be estimated by identifying the scoring elements which are present on each of the three molars in a jaw, and adding together the weights associated with each such element.

Tooth wear is necessarily only an approximate means of assessing age: it is clearly possible for an individual animal to have teeth which are more worn, in every respect, than a 'typical' animal some years older. Nevertheless, it was found that, in a sample of 119 known-aged (tagged at birth) Red deer from the island of Rum, the majority of those under 15 years were accurately aged to within 4 months (the scheme is not successful in distinguishing between animals older than 15 years, by which point the teeth are fully worn). While this is sufficiently accurate for most ageing purposes, it clearly does not provide a useful assessment of seasonality.

The scoring scheme as it stands relies on the existence of a complete jaw (or at least on all three molars), but could easily be adapted to enable ageing to be carried out (perhaps with some loss of accuracy) using a single molar. It should be noted, however, that it can be hard to distinguish between isolated first and second molars. The method by which the scheme is derived, described in Chapter 6 and Appendix 4, could equally be used to obtain similar schemes for Red deer from different environments, and for other species.

Obvious advantages of the scoring scheme as a method of age estimation are that it is easy to learn and use, requires no specialised equipment, and does not involve the destruction of the sample. Moreover, in contrast to incremental analysis, the technique is highly reliable: that is, an examiner can reliably obtain the same estimated age when scoring a jaw on two different occasions, as can two examiners scoring the same jaw independently. The statistical basis of reliability studies, and the reliability analysis for the scoring scheme, are presented in Chapter 7. The individual reliabilities of two different examiners and the interexaminer reliability between these two examiners are all found to be 97% or greater. This means that if the two examiners score a large collection of jaws, the variation of the scores obtained due to examiner unreliability and differences between the two examiners will be less than 3% of the total variation of scores obtained.

In conclusion, the scoring scheme is substantially more accurate and reliable than cementum incremental analysis as a means of age estimation, and has the additional advantages of being quicker, cheaper, and non-destructive. I therefore recommend strongly that the scoring scheme be used to build up age profiles of archaeological populations until such a time as significant advances have been made in the understanding of incremental structures and the ability of researchers to make accurate and reliable age estimates using incremental analysis.

4. SUGGESTIONS FOR FURTHER RESEARCH

A great deal of further research is required on cementum incremental analysis before it is sufficiently well understood to be a useful tool in an archaeological context. One of the first priorities must be to attempt to understand the causes of incremental structures in cementum. This is a difficult undertaking for two reasons: first, because the incremental structures are very complex; and second, because they may be affected by several different life events, each of which impacts upon several different causal factors. Thus it is important to devise experiments which isolate single causal factors as much as possible (as in Lieberman 1993). It is therefore necessary to study animals whose life histories are known. Ideally, one would make use of detectable dyes with animals which are kept under carefully controlled conditions over a long period of time. It should also be borne in mind that incremental structures are species-dependent, so that such experiments should be carried out for each species which one wishes to study. A detailed study of the differences in incremental structures between male and female animals would also be worthwhile, particularly if they are influenced by hormonal factors.

In order to apply cementum incremental analysis to archaeological specimens, it is also important to understand how the incremental structure may be damaged or modified by prolonged exposure. A possible experiment would be to section teeth from one side of each of a sample of jaws, and to bury the other sides in varying conditions for varying time periods before excavating them and sectioning them. Taphonomic effects on isolated teeth and on tooth fragments could also be studied in this way.

More routine and short-term research could be carried out by adapting the scoring scheme to other species, to Red deer from other environments, and to isolated teeth.

5. IMPLICATIONS FOR STUDIES OF PREHISTORY

As has already been discussed, the principal conclusions of this thesis concerning the application of cementum incremental analysis in the archaeological context are negative: incremental structures are not at present sufficiently well understood, or sufficiently well correlated with basic events in an animal's life, to justify the use of this destructive technique on valuable archaeological material. A number of researchers have attempted to analyse archaeological teeth, or fragments of archaeological teeth, using this technique. Given both the unreliability and the inherent problems with incremental analysis which have been described in this thesis, it must be questioned whether any insights into human prehistory have been obtained which justify the destruction of samples. As I have already explained, this is not to suggest that archaeologists should not be studying incremental analysis with a view to its eventual application to archaeological material: if in the course of time it becomes possible to understand which basic events in an animal's life are reflected in the incremental structure of its cementum, and to establish that the incremental structure is not unduly influenced by taphonomic considerations, then incremental analysis will become a powerful and valuable tool in the study of prehistory. For example, if it were possible to identify nutritional stress in animals from their dental cementum, this would give insights into both environmental conditions and hunting strategies in prehistory.

The positive results presented in this thesis concern the development of a new scoring scheme by means of which it is possible to estimate the age of Red deer on the basis of tooth wear. Scoring schemes are a familiar tool of archaeologists, but I believe that the one presented here, by virtue of the range of scoring elements identified and the techniques used to optimise the weights associated to the elements, is highly accurate and repeatable.

The study of the reliability of the scoring scheme is, so far as I know, new in this context, and has most encouraging results. I would suggest that this technique should be applied to other standard archaeological methods (such as pollen analysis) in which an element of subjectivity is involved, or there is a possibility of observer error. It should be stressed that a method is only useful if it is both accurate and reliable. Moreover, knowing the reliability of a method makes it possible to determine how many times a measurement should be made independently before one can be confident of its correctness.

Because of the wide range of factors which can influence tooth wear, this method cannot allow the determination of seasonality once eruption is complete. However, it does make it possible to build up age profiles, which in turn give valuable information about hunting practice. In particular, if the majority of animals killed are either very young or very old, it suggests that hunters were content to make the easiest kills they could; whereas the presence of cull patterns suggests herd management. If different hunting practices can be established for neighbouring groups, this can also give information about the movement and interaction of these groups.

As presented here, the scoring scheme is applicable to Red deer from a highland environment: however, the methods used in its derivation are quite general. I would therefore recommend the extension of the scheme to other environments and to other species, in order to provide a working database for archaeologists.

Appendices

1. Terminology

Acellular cementum:	Cementum which does not contain entrapped cementoblasts
Afibrillar:	Contains no collagen fibres
Alveoli:	Bone socket in the jaw bone
Anterior:	In front - see Mesial
Apex:	The bottom point of the tooth's root
Apical:	Pertaining to the apex
Apposition:	Addition to a surface
Appositional rate:	Speed of deposition
Attrition:	In dental terms, tooth wear
Banding:	Layers of cementum separated by lines
Buccal:	Cheek side
Canaliculi:	Bone like material coating the root of a tooth
Cementoblasts:	Cubic cells forming a single layer in contact with the dentine
Cementocytes:	Cementoblasts which have ceased to form cementum
Cementogenesis:	The process of cementum formation
Cementoid:	A thin layer of unmineralised cementum
Cementum:	A pale yellow, bone like material which covers the entire root
Cervid:	Deer
Collagen:	A fibrous protein, found in dentine, cement and bone
Coronal End:	The top of the tooth's crown
Crown:	The area of tooth covered by enamel projecting in to the mouth (see Enamel)
Cusp:	Mounds of enamel
Cytology:	Concerned with cells
Decalcification:	Removal of mineral component of tooth or bone
Deciduous Teeth:	First or Primary teeth which are replaced by Permanent teeth as the animal ages
Dentine:	The majority of the substance of a tooth
Dentition:	The relationship of the teeth to each other
Enamel:	A hard crystalline tissue coating the crown of a tooth (see Crown)
Encapsulation:	Embedding in resin
Eruption:	Movement of forming and formed tooth through bone in to the mouth
Exothermic:	Chemical reaction that raises the temperature of the components
Extrinsic Fibres:	(Sharpey's fibres) Fibres formed outside the cementum which run perpendicular to the root surface
Hypoconulid:	Most posterior cusp of mandibular third molar
Increment:	A layer or band of cementum
Infundibula:	Infoldings within the body of the tooth's crown
Interradicular area:	Area between the roots of multi-rooted teeth – sometimes called pad cementum
Intrinsic Fibres:	Fibres formed by the cementoblasts which run parallel to the root surface
Mandible:	The lower jaw
Maxilla:	The upper jaw
Mesial:	Anterior aspect of tooth
Micron:	A measurement - 1/1000 of a millimetre
Microtome:	A machine for slicing thin sections of tissue
Neonatal:	At birth
Occlusal Surface:	Biting surface of a tooth
Occlusion:	The relationship of the upper and lower teeth to each other
Ossification:	The mineralisation of bone
Osteoporosis:	The pitting of long bones in birds and mammals
Periodontal Ligament:	Flexible fibres which attach the tooth to the surrounding bone
Precement:	The organic matrix of cementum before it becomes mineralised
Proteoglycans:	Organic protein - part of the cementum organic matrix
Pulp Chamber:	Area in the middle of the root surrounded by dentine
Quiescence:	Inactive
Resorption:	The removal of mineralised tooth or bone by resorbing cells
Root:	The portion of a tooth covered by cementum

Appendix 2: Work sheet for microscopical examination of bands and lines in cementum

Date:

Section number:

Identification code:

Observer:

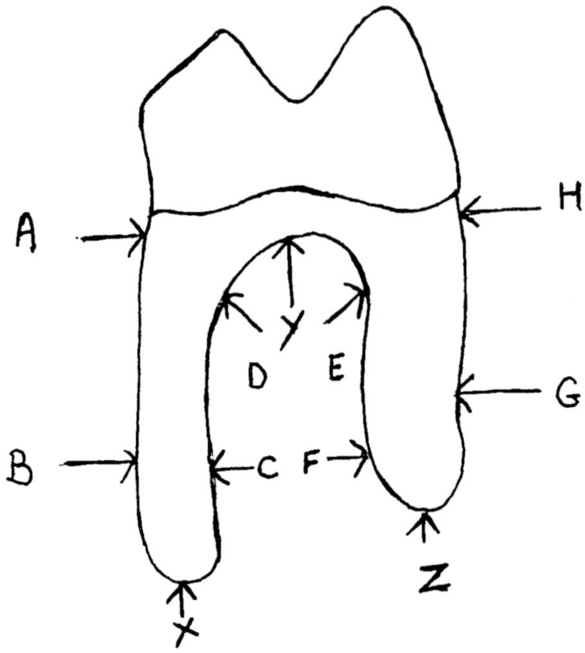

Layers				
	Bands	**Lines**	**Magnification**	**Outer edge band/line**
A				
B				
C				
D				
E				
F				
G				
H				
X				
Y				
Z				

Appendix 3: Scoring worksheet

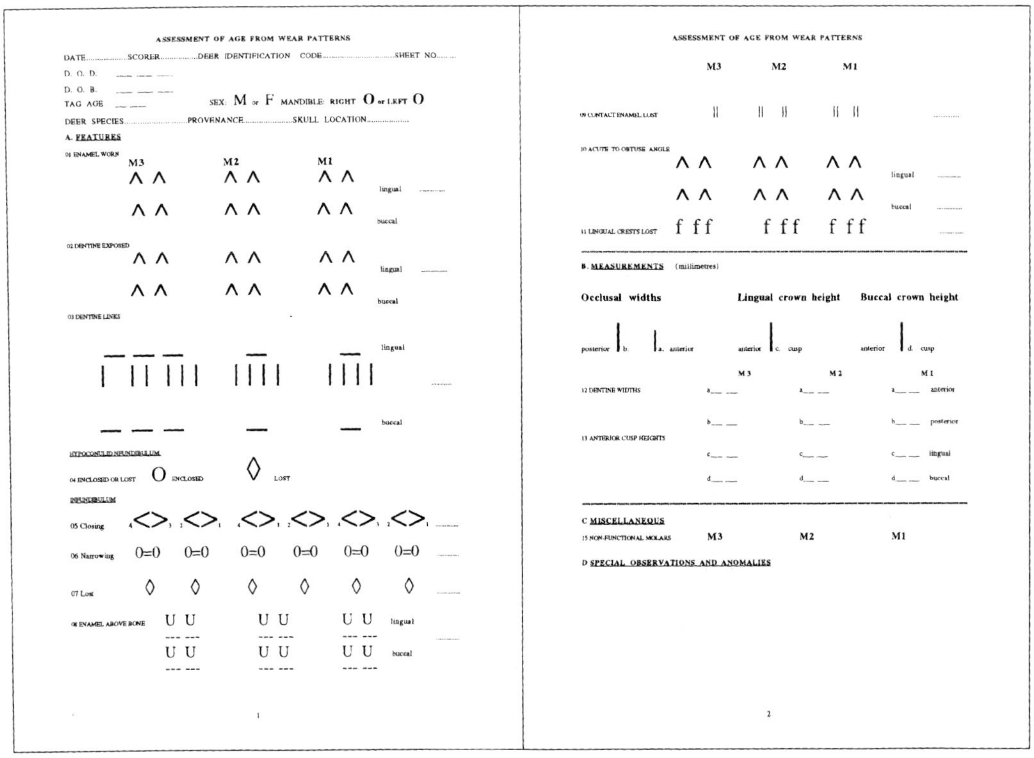

Appendix 4: Derivation of the Scoring Scheme

In this appendix, the steps which were used to derive the scoring scheme described in chapter 6 are described in detail. The aim is twofold: first, to clarify by means of example the method adopted; and second, to provide a model for the derivation of other similar schemes, perhaps for a different species, or for red deer from a different environment, for which tooth wear may proceed more or less rapidly.

For reasons of space, and for the sake of clarity, the data used in this appendix is fictitious. It will be assumed that a sample of ten known-aged jaws is available, and that six distinct scoring elements have been identified: these six elements will be called Sc1, Sc2, Sc3, Sc4, Sc5, and Sc6. Of course, in attempting to derive a real scoring scheme it would be desirable to have a much larger sample, and to identify more than six scoring elements: the method, however, would be identical.

Microsoft's Excel spreadsheet has been used to carry out these calculations.

Step 1: Data Entry

Having scored each of the six scoring elements on each of the ten jaws, this data is entered into an empty spreadsheet, as shown below

STEP1.XLS

	A	B	C	D	E	F	G	H
1	Jaw No.	True Age	Sc1	Sc2	Sc3	Sc4	Sc5	Sc6
2	1	59	5	4	7	4	3	5
3	2	66	6	4	8	4	3	6
4	3	62	6	4	8	4	3	6
5	4	48	4	3	6	3	3	5
6	5	12	1	0	2	0	0	2
7	6	30	2	2	4	2	3	4
8	7	35	5	3	2	1	1	4
9	8	24	4	4	2	1	1	4
10	9	31	4	3	3	2	3	4
11	10	42	6	4	4	3	3	5

The known age in months of each jaw has been entered, together with the score which was assigned to it for each of the six scoring elements identified. The aim of the following calculations is to identify six *weights*, one for each scoring element, such that when the scores for each element are multiplied by their weights and added together, the result is as close as possible to the known age of the jaw.

Step 2: Entering formulae for the estimated age and errors

The spreadsheet should now be extended to enable weights to be assigned to each scoring element, and to calculate the estimated age of each jaw on the basis of these weights, and the difference between the estimated age and the known age.

STEP2XLS

	A	B	C	D	E	F	G	H	I	J
1	Jaw No.	True Age	Sc1	Sc2	Sc3	Sc4	Sc5	Sc6	Estimated Age	Error
2	1	59	5	4	7	4	3	5	23	36
3	2	66	6	4	8	4	3	6	25	41
4	3	62	6	4	8	4	3	6	25	37
5	4	48	4	3	6	3	3	5	19	29
6	5	12	1	0	2	0	0	2	3	9
7	6	30	2	2	4	2	3	4	13	17
8	7	35	5	3	2	1	1	4	12	23
9	8	24	4	4	2	1	1	4	12	12
10	9	31	4	3	3	2	3	4	15	16
11	10	42	6	4	4	3	3	5	20	22
12										
13		Weights	1	1	1	1	1	1		
14		Constant	0							
15										
16		Total Error	201							

In rows 13 and 14 of this spreadsheet, an initial choice of weights for each scoring element, and of a constant, which will be added to the estimated age at the end of the calculation has been made. The particular values chosen here are of no importance - the spreadsheet will later adjust them in order to get the best possible match between the known ages and the estimated ages of the jaws.

The data in the other new rows and columns has not been entered by hand, but has been calculated by the spreadsheet. Column I contains the estimated ages of the ten jaws, as calculated using the weights and constant in rows 13 and 14, and column J gives the error for each jaw: the discrepancy between the true age and the estimated age. The formulae which have been used to calculate these values are shown below:

STEP2XLS

	I	J
1	Estimated Age	Error
2	=C$14+C2*C$13+D2*D$13+E2*E$13+F2*F$13+G2*G$13+H2*H$14	=ABS(B2-I2)
3	=C$14+C3*C$13+D3*D$13+E3*E$13+F3*F$13+G3*G$13+H3*H$14	=ABS(B3-I3)
4	=C$14+C4*C$13+D4*D$13+E4*E$13+F4*F$13+G4*G$13+H4*H$14	=ABS(B4-I4)
5	=C$14+C5*C$13+D5*D$13+E5*E$13+F5*F$13+G5*G$13+H5*H$14	=ABS(B5-I5)
6	=C$14+C6*C$13+D6*D$13+E6*E$13+F6*F$13+G6*G$13+H6*H$14	=ABS(B6-I6)
7	=C$14+C7*C$13+D7*D$13+E7*E$13+F7*F$13+G7*G$13+H7*H$14	=ABS(B7-I7)
8	=C$14+C8*C$13+D8*D$13+E8*E$13+F8*F$13+G8*G$13+H8*H$14	=ABS(B8-I8)
9	=C$14+C9*C$13+D9*D$13+E9*E$13+F9*F$13+G9*G$13+H9*H$14	=ABS(B9-I9)
10	=C$14+C10*C$13+D10*D$13+E10*E$13+F10*F$13+G10*G$13+H10	=ABS(B10-I1
11	=C$14+C11*C$13+D11*D$13+E11*E$13+F11*F$13+G11*G$13+H11	=ABS(B11-I1

The formula in cell I2 tells the spreadsheet to fill this cell with the value of cell C14 (the constant), plus the value of C2 times that of C13 (the first scoring element times its weight), plus the value of D2 times that of D13 (the second scoring element times its weight), and so on for the other four scoring elements. Once this formula has been entered into I2, it can be 'dragged' down the rest of the column, with the spreadsheet automatically adjusting the relevant parts of each formula so as to refer to each jaw in turn.

The formula in cell J2 tells the spreadsheet to fill this cell with the *absolute value* of the difference between the contents of B2 (the true age of the first jaw) and the contents of I2 (the estimated age). The effect of the ABS is to ensure that this number is always greater than or equal to zero, regardless of whether the true age or the estimated age is greater. Once again, it is only necessary to enter this formula in J2, and it can then be dragged down into cells J3 to J11, with the relevant parts of the formula being automatically adjusted.

Finally, cell C16 contains the total error, taken over all of the jaws in the sample. The formula entered into this cell is
=SUM(J2:J11)-LARGE(J2:J11,1)

The first part of this formula simply adds together the contents of cells J2 to J11: that is, the errors in the age estimations of the ten jaws. To understand the second part of the formula, remember that it was decided that the scoring scheme should allow for the possibility of observer error or very unusual jaws by ignoring a certain number of 'outlying' data points. The function LARGE(J2:J11,1) returns the largest of the values of the cells between J2 and J11 (in this case 41), and this value is subtracted from the sum: thus the largest of the ten errors is effectively ignored, and cell C16 contains the total of the other nine errors. With a sample of only ten jaws, no more than one such score should be attributed to an outlier: however in the real scoring scheme, where a sample of 41 jaws was used, the largest four errors were all ignored.

Notice that the total error is very large: this is because the weights have not been chosen sensibly. The final step is to get the spreadsheet to determine what choice of weights should be made in order to make the total error as small as possible.

Step 3: Determining the weights

The aim, then, is to adjust the weights and the constant (that is, the contents of cells C13 to H13 and cell C14), in such a way as to make the total error (that is, the contents of cell C16) as small as possible. Also, in order that the scoring scheme should be straightforward to apply in practice, it is required that the weights and the constant should take on whole number values.

Microsoft Excel provides a 'solver' feature which automates this type of calculation. The following figure shows how the solver dialog box should be set up in this case:

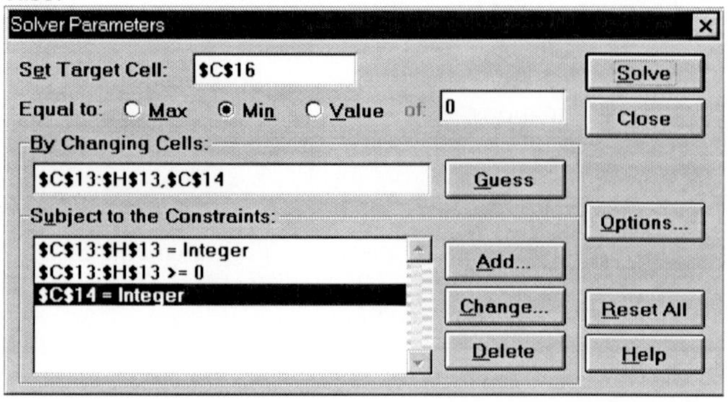

The *Target Cell* has been set to cell C16, the total error: this is the cell whose value we would like to make as small as possible. The fact that this is our aim is signalled by the choice of the *Min* radio button, which requests the spreadsheet to minimise the contents of this cell. The cells which the spreadsheet is permitted to change in order to effect this minimisation are given in the *By Changing Cells* text box: cells C13 to H13 (the weights) and cell C14 (the constant) may be changed. Finally, the *Subject to the Constraints* input box tells the spreadsheet what sort of changes it is permitted to make: the weights must remain integers (whole numbers); the weights must be greater than or equal to zero; and the constant must remain an integer.

Clicking the *Solve* button causes Excel to carry out the minimisation. In this case, the process takes about 15 seconds, but for the real scoring scheme, where much more data is involved, the minimisation takes several hours. Once the calculation is complete, the spreadsheet is automatically updated to reflect the best possible choices of weights and constants.

STEP3.XLS

	A	B	C	D	E	F	G	H	I	J
1	Jaw No.	True Age	Sc1	Sc2	Sc3	Sc4	Sc5	Sc6	Estimated Age	Error
2	1	59	5	4	7	4	3	5	57	2
3	2	66	6	4	8	4	3	6	64	2
4	3	62	6	4	8	4	3	6	64	2
5	4	48	4	3	6	3	3	5	47	1
6	5	12	1	0	2	0	0	2	12	0
7	6	30	2	2	4	2	3	4	30	0
8	7	35	5	3	2	1	1	4	25	10
9	8	24	4	4	2	1	1	4	24	0
10	9	31	4	3	3	2	3	4	30	1
11	10	42	6	4	4	3	3	5	42	0
12										
13		Weights	2	1	5	2	0	2		
14		Constant	0							
15										
16		Total Erro	8							

Thus the best possible choice of weights for the six scoring elements are 2, 1, 5, 2, 0, and 2 respectively: scoring element 5 is seen to be irrelevant to the final age estimation. In this case, no constant should be added to the final score obtained. Thus, in order to estimate the age of a jaw, one should add up twice element 1, element 2, five times element 3, two times element 4, and two times element 6. The estimated ages resulting from this scheme are automatically displayed in column I, and the associated errors in column J are updated.

Notice that the largest error is for jaw number 7, and that this outlier has been ignored in the determination of the total error. An error might have been made in scoring this jaw or in recording its known age, or the animal concerned may have been subject to some condition which made the rate of wear of its teeth atypical.

As was emphasised in chapter 6, the accuracy of this scoring scheme is unconfirmed until it has been tested on a second known age sample, unrelated to the one which was used to determine the weights.

APPENDIX 5: A QUICK GUIDE TO RELIABILITY CALCULATION

In Chapter 7, the reliability of the scoring scheme for age estimation was assessed: the statistical basis of the reliability analysis was described, and the actual data pertaining to the scoring by two examiners of a sample of 53 jaws was analysed. The aim of this Appendix is to present the techniques involved in the analysis in a way which is hopefully more accessible to a non-mathematical reader. To this end, the data set used is fictitious, being smaller and simpler than the real data which was considered in Chapter 7. It is undeniable that a reliability analysis involves a long sequence of calculations: however, these calculations involve nothing more complicated than simple arithmetic operations, which although tedious to carry out by hand, can easily be automated using a spreadsheet program.

Intraexaminer reliability

Suppose that a single examiner scores each of a collection of jaws a number of times. For the sake of this example, suppose that he scores 10 jaws 3 times each. The aim is to estimate the reliability with which he can arrive at the same score when he studies a given jaw independently on separate occasions.

Step 1

Draw up a table giving the scores recorded. The data given below is fictitious.

Jaw No.	Score 1	Score 2	Score 3
1	92	95	86
2	113	101	112
3	65	64	64
4	131	124	129
5	36	36	33
6	67	65	50
7	84	91	92
8	103	97	95
9	52	49	46
10	29	31	30

Step 2

Work out the average of all the scores recorded. In this case, add up the 30 scores to get a total of 2262, and divide by 30 to get the average of 75.4.

Step 3

Append a column to the table giving the average score recorded for each jaw. For example, the average score for jaw number 1 is obtained by adding 92, 95, and 86 to get 273, and divide by 3 to give 91.

Jaw No.	Score 1	Score 2	Score 3	Average
1	92	95	86	91
2	113	101	112	108.6666
3	65	64	64	64.33333
4	131	124	129	128
5	36	36	33	35
6	67	65	50	60.66666
7	84	91	92	89
8	103	97	95	98.33333
9	52	49	46	49
10	29	31	30	30

Step 4

Now calculate another column, given by subtracting each of the three scores for a given jaw from the average for that jaw in turn, squaring the results (i.e. multiplying them by themselves), adding the three numbers which result, and dividing the total by one less than the number of measurements on the jaw (in this case, 2). Thus, for the first jaw, subtracting 92, 95, and 86 from 91 gives -1, -4, and 5. Squaring these numbers gives 1, 16, and 25. Adding the results gives 1+16+25=42, and dividing by 2 gives 21. This number is called the *sample variance* of the three scores. Notice that larger variances occur when the three scores for the given jaw vary substantially.

Jaw No.	Score 1	Score 2	Score 3	Average	Variance
1	92	95	86	91	21
2	113	101	112	108.6666	44.33333
3	65	64	64	64.33333	0.333333
4	131	124	129	128	13
5	36	36	33	35	3
6	67	65	50	60.66666	86.33333
7	84	91	92	89	19
8	103	97	95	98.33333	17.33333
9	52	49	46	49	9
10	29	31	30	30	1

Step 5

The *Within subjects mean square* or *WMS* can now be calculated, as the average of the 10 variances. In this case, the WMS is obtained by adding the 10 values in the final column of the table above, to give 214.3333, and dividing by 10 to give 21.43333. This value gives a measure of the variation of the data due to examiner error.

Step 6

Now, for each jaw, subtract the average score from the overall average score of 75.4 obtained in step 2, and square the result. Thus for jaw number 1, subtract 91 from 75.4 to get -15.6, and square the result to get 243.36. For jaw number 2, subtract 108.6666 from 75.4 to obtain -33.2667, and square the result to get 1106.671. Repeat this procedure for each of the ten jaws, and put the results in a seventh column:

Jaw No.	Score 1	Score 2	Score 3	Average	Variance	Ov Av-Av Sq
1	92	95	86	91	21	243.36
2	113	101	112	108.6666	44.33333	1106.671
3	65	64	64	64.33333	0.333333	122.4711
4	131	124	129	128	13	2766.76
5	36	36	33	35	3	1632.16
6	67	65	50	60.66666	86.33333	217.0711
7	84	91	92	89	19	184.96
8	103	97	95	98.33333	17.33333	525.9377
9	52	49	46	49	9	696.96
10	29	31	30	30	1	2061.16

Step 7

The *Between subjects mean square* or *BMS* can now be calculated. Add together the values in the final column of the table, multiply by the number of measurements on each jaw (here 3), and divide by one fewer than the number of jaws (here 9). In this case, the total of the values in the final column is 9557.511, so on multiplying by 3 and dividing by 9 the BMS is found to be 3185.837.

Step 8

The reliability can now be estimated. To do this, first subtract the WMS from the BMS: this gives a value of 3185.837-21.433=3164.404. Next multiply the WMS by one fewer than the number of measurements on each jaw (here 2) to get 21.433 x 2 = 42.866. Add this number to the BMS to get 3185.837+42.866=3228.703. Finally, divide the number 3164.404 in the first part of the calculation by the number 3228.703 just obtained to get 3164.404 ÷ 3228.703=0.980. This is the estimated value of the reliability.

Interexaminer reliability

Now suppose that each of a number of examiners scores the same collection of jaws. For the sake of the example here, suppose that two examiners each score each of 10 jaws. The aim here is twofold: first, to decide whether there is evidence to reject the hypothesis that the two examiners are scoring in the same way; and second, to estimate the reliability of scores obtained on a collection of jaws each of which is scored by only one of the two examiners, chosen randomly. The calculations are no more difficult than in the study of intraexaminer reliability, but are a little more complicated.

Step 1

Draw up a table giving the scores obtained by each of the two examiners on each jaw

Jaw No.	Exam 1	Exam 2
1	53	60
2	98	103
3	77	75
4	45	51
5	103	112
6	134	134
7	27	29
8	61	70
9	83	80
10	71	73

Step 2

Work out the average of the scores obtained by each examiner, and of all 20 scores obtained by the two examiners together. In this case, the average score of examiner 1 is 75.2, the average score of examiner 2 is 78.7, and the overall average is 76.95.

Step 3

For each jaw, subtract the overall average 76.95 from the score obtained by examiner 1, and square the result. Thus, for jaw 1, subtract 76.95 from 53 to get -23.95, and square this number to get 573.6025. Tabulate these values in a fourth column of the table. Do the same for examiner 2, and tabulate the results in the fifth column. For example, the first entry in the fifth column is obtained by subtracting 76.95 from 60 to get -16.95, and squaring the result to get 287.3025.

Jaw No.	Exam 1	Exam 2	Ex1-Av Sq	Ex2-Av Sq
1	53	60	573.6025	287.3025
2	98	103	443.1025	678.6025
3	77	75	0.0025	3.8025
4	45	51	1020.802	673.4025
5	103	112	678.6025	1228.502
6	134	134	3254.702	3254.702
7	27	29	2495.002	2299.202
8	61	70	254.4025	48.3025
9	83	80	36.6025	9.3025
10	71	73	35.4025	15.6025

Step 4

Estimate the *total variance* by adding together the 20 values in the final two columns of the above table, and dividing by one fewer than the number of values (here 19). In this example, adding the 20 values gives 17290.95, and dividing by 19 gives 910.05 as an estimate of the total variance.

Step 5

For each jaw, calculate the average of the scores obtained by the two examiners for that jaw (so for jaw 1, the average is half of 53+60, or 56.5). These values are tabulated in the sixth column below. Subtract the overall average 76.95, obtained in step 2, from each of these values, and square the result. Thus for jaw 1, the value is obtained by subtracting 76.95 from 56.5 to give -20.45, and squaring this number to give 418.2025. These values are given in the seventh column below.

Jaw No.	Exam 1	Exam 2	Ex1-Av Sq	Ex2-Av Sq	Average	Av-Ov Av Sq
1	53	60	573.6025	287.3025	56.5	418.2025
2	98	103	443.1025	678.6025	100.5	554.6025
3	77	75	0.0025	3.8025	76	0.9025
4	45	51	1020.802	673.4025	48	838.1025
5	103	112	678.6025	1228.502	107.5	933.3025
6	134	134	3254.702	3254.702	134	3254.702
7	27	29	2495.002	2299.202	28	2396.102
8	61	70	254.4025	48.3025	65.5	131.1025
9	83	80	36.6025	9.3025	81.5	20.7025
10	71	73	35.4025	15.6025	72	24.5025

Step 6

The *Jaw mean square* or *JMS* can now be calculated by adding together the values in the final column of the table above, multiplying by 2, and dividing by one fewer than the number of jaws (here 9). Adding the values gives a total of 8572.225, which on multiplying by 2 and dividing by 9 gives a value of 1904.939 for the JMS.

Step 7

The *Scorer mean square* or *SMS* is calculated by subtracting the overall average score 76.95 from each examiner's individual average, squaring the two numbers obtained, adding together the squares, and multiplying by the number of jaws in the sample. In this case, the first examiner's average is 75.2. Subtracting 76.95 from this gives -1.75, which on squaring gives 3.0625. Carrying out the same calculation with the second examiner gives the same result 3.0625 (as it always will when there are only two examiners). Adding 3.0625 to 3.0625 and multiplying by 10 (the number of jaws) gives a value of 61.25 for the SMS.

Step 8

Finally, calculate the *Error mean square* or *EMS*. To do this, multiply the total variance 910.05 (step 4) by one fewer than twice the number of jaws scored (here 19). Subtract from this the JMS 1904.939 multiplied by one fewer than the number of jaws scored (here 9). Finally subtract the SMS 61.25, and divide the result by one fewer than the number of jaws scored (here 9). In this example, the calculation gives (19 x 910.05) - (9 x 1904.939) - 61.25 = 85.249, which when divided by 9 gives a value of 9.472 for the EMS.

Step 9

To test the hypothesis that the scorers are scoring in the same way, the ratio SMS/EMS must be compared to tabulated values of the F distribution with 1 and 9 degrees of freedom (9 being one fewer than the number of jaws in the sample). In this case, SMS divided by EMS is 6.466 (this says that the variation in the data due to differences between the scorers is about 6 times the variation due to scorer error). To test whether there is evidence to reject the hypothesis of same scoring technique at a 95% level of significance, compare this value to $F_{1,9,0.05}$, which is given in statistical tables as 5.117. Since 6.466 is greater than 5.117, there is evidence to reject the hypothesis at a 95% level of significance (i.e., when we allow a 1 in 20 probability of rejecting the hypothesis when it is in fact true). On the other hand, $F_{1,9,0.01}$ is equal to 10.562, so there is no evidence to reject the hypothesis at a 99% level of significance (i.e., when we only allow a 1 in 100 probability of rejecting the hypothesis when it is in fact true).

Step 10

Finally, to estimate the reliability of joint measurements by the two examiners: first subtract the EMS from the JMS and multiply the result by the number of jaws. This gives 10 x (1904.939-9.472), or 18954.67. Then calculate the number of jaws times the JMS, plus the SMS, plus one fewer than the number of jaws times the EMS. This gives (10 x 1904.939) + 61.25 + (9 x 9.472) or 19195.89. The joint reliability is estimated by dividing the first result by the second: 18954.67□19195.89=0.987. Thus the joint reliability is good, despite the fact that there are significant differences between the two examiners: this is because the variations due to differences between the examiners are small compared to variations due to differences between the jaws.

Appendix 6: Thin section data and analysis

In Chapter 4, thin sections of first molars of fourteen known-aged (tagged at birth) Red deer are discussed in detail. It is shown there: first, that the number of layers varies substantially at different locations around a given section; second, that at no individual location is this number consistently close to the age in years of the animal; and third, that the outer layer also typically varies around each section, and does not give any consistent guide to season of death. This appendix provides details of a sample of 120 sections, each of which was examined at each of eleven standard locations. The sample includes the 14 known-aged sections discussed in Chapter 4, a further 20 whose ages were estimated by experienced stalkers on the basis of tooth wear and body weight, and 86 of unknown age. The animals come from a variety of locations in England and Scotland, and comprise 84 males, 23 females, and 13 of unknown sex.

As explained in Chapter 4, a larger sample of jaws of known age was available (and was used to derive the scoring scheme), but it was decided that the remainder of this valuable collection should not be sectioned, since it was apparent that no reasonable age or seasonality assessment could be made on the basis of thin sections. The data presented here supports that decision: it will be seen that there is almost always a substantial discrepancy between the number of layers visible at different locations around the tooth root, and that the number of layers observed does not correlate well with the age in years, either known or estimated, of the animal being studied.

The data obtained from the sections is given in Table 13. The columns of this table show, from left to right:

- The slide number, which was assigned upon obtaining a successful section. The known-aged collection is numbered from 501 to 514.
- The provenance of the animal: Aber (Abernethy), Woll (Wollaton), Worm (Wormsley), Eust (Euston), Bal (Balmoral), Str (StrathVaich), BAr (Ben Arnine), CM (Creag Meagadih), or High (unknown Highland provenance).
- The month of the year in which the animal died. With the exception of the known aged sample, these months tend to be concentrated in the English and Scottish hunting seasons.
- The sex of the animal: U indicates that the sex is unknown.
- The estimated age of the animal at death, if available. For the known-aged sample, this column contains the known age at death in years and months.
- The tooth which was sectioned. In the few cases where this is not M1, the tooth was from an animal whose M1 was also sectioned.
- The remaining 11 columns contain the number of bands, and of lines, observed at each of the 11 standard locations indicated in Appendix 2. The symbol U indicates that the section was unreadable at that location (in that it was impossible to distinguish accurately the bands and lines), and D that the tooth was damaged in such a way as to make any attempt to read the section pointless.

No	*Prov*	*Mth*	*S*	*Est*	*Tth*	*A*	*B*	*C*	*D*	*E*	*F*	*G*	*H*	*X*	*Y*	*Z*
1	Aber	10	M		M1	3/4	2/3	2/3	U	3/3	2/3	U	U	1/2	5/5	U
2	Aber	10	M		M1	2/2	2/1	2/1	3/2	4/3	1/1	3/2	3/2	U	5/4	5/4
3	Aber	10	M		M1	1/0	1/0	U	4/3	2/1	1/0	U	U	4/3	U	U
4	Aber	10	M		M1	U	1/0	2/1	3/3	2/1	U	2/1	2/1	U	U	4/4
5	Aber	2	F		M1	3/3	U	U	U	1/1	4/3	2/2	2/2	D	U	U
6	Aber	12	M		M1	1/1	2/1	1/1	1/1	2/2	2/1	2/2	2/3	U	5/4	U
7	Aber	10	M		M1	2/2	2/2	D	D	1/1	1/1	U	1/0	U	U	U
8	Aber	12	M		M1	1/0	1/1	1/0	5/5	2/1	1/0	1/1	2/1	U	U	U
9	Aber	12	F		M1	2/1	1/1	2/1	4/4	1/0	2/2	2/2	4/4	U	U	U
10	Aber	10	M		M1	4/3	2/2	D	D	U	U	U	U	U	U	U
11	Aber	10	M		M1	2/1	U	2/1	1/0	1/0	U	2/3	U	U	3/2	U
12	Aber	10	M		M1	2/2	2/1	3/2	4/3	2/2	U	2/2	4/3	U	U	U
14	Aber	1	F		M1	2/2	D	2/3	3/2	1/2	U	2/1	3/3	U	4/3	4/3
15	Aber	12	M		M1	3/2	5/4	4/3	3/3	5/5	5/4	3/2	5/5	U	U	U
16	Aber	12	F	10+	M1	1/0	U	U	U	3/4	5/4	1/0	2/1	U	U	U
17	Aber	10	M		M1	2/1	5/4	5/5	3/2	7/6	7/7	5/4	2/1	U	U	U
18	Aber	1	F		M1	2/1	2/1	U	3/3	U	2/1	U	2/1	U	10/9	U
19	Aber	10	M	1	M1	U	2/1	2/2	2/2	U	3/2	U	3/3	U	U	U
20	Aber	10	M	6-7	M1	1/0	2/1	2/1	1/0	U	1/1	2/1	3/2	U	5/5	3/3
21	Aber	10	M		M1	1/0	U	2/1	1/0	U	2/1	U	1/0	U	2/1	U
22	Aber	10	M		M1	1/0	2/1	5/6	2/1	1/0	U	1/1	U	U	1/0	U
23	Aber	10	M		M1	1/0	1/0	1/0	1/1	1/1	1/0	1/0	1/0	U	1/0	U
24	Aber	12	M		M1	2/1	2/1	1/1	1/0	4/3	1/0	2/1	2/1	7/6	U	U
25	Aber	10	M	2	M1	2/1	2/1	2/1	2/2	2/1	1/0	2/1	U	U	U	U
26	Aber	10	M	3-4	M1	2/1	2/1	2/1	2/1	3/3	2/1	3/2	2/1	U	U	U
27	Aber	10	M		M1	U	U	U	U	3/2	3/2	2/2	2/1	3/3	4/4	3/3
28	Aber	10	M		M1	2/2	1/1	1/0	1/1	2/1	2/1	3/2	2/1	U	4/3	U
29	Aber	10	M		M1	3/2	2/1	D	D	1/0	1/0	2/1	2/2	4/3	3/2	3/2
30	Aber	10	M		M1	4/3	5/4	5/5	3/2	2/2	2/2	3/3	2/1	U	5/5	6/5
31	Aber	10	M		M1	6/5	3/2	1/0	U	U	2/2	U	3/2	4/4	3/3	4/3
32	Aber	10	M		M1	1/0	4/3	2/1	4/3	3/3	5/4	3/2	5/4	2/2	U	U
33	Aber	12	F		M1	2/1	2/1	2/1	1/1	U	10/10	U	3/2	U	5/5	U
34	Aber	12	F	3	M1	2/1	2/1	2/1	2/2	2/1	2/2	2/1	2/1	U	2/2	2/1
35	Aber	10	M	8-9	M1	4/3	U	U	1/0	6/5	5/4	8/7	8/7	7/7	7/6	5/4
36	Aber	12	M		M1	3/2	U	U	U	2/1	3/3	2/1	3/2	2/2	2/2	2/2
38	Aber	10	M		M1	3/2	2/1	D	D	U	U	U	U	U	U	U
40	Woll	11	M		M1	2/2	2/1	U	U	1/1	2/1	U	U	U	U	D
41	Woll	11	M		M1	1/1	1/1	1/1	U	2/1	U	1/1	2/1	U	U	U
42	Woll	11	M		M1	D	D	2/1	D	1/0	1/0	1/1	2/2	U	U	U
43	Woll	11	M	1	M1	4/3	2/1	1/0	1/0	3/2	3/3	4/3	3/2	4/4	4/4	4/4
45	Woll	11	M		M1	1/0	1/0	2/1	U	U	U	2/1	1/0	U	U	U
49	Worm	11	M		M2	2/1	1/0	2/1	2/2	3/2	3/2	D	2/1	2/2	3/2	2/2
50	Worm	11	M		M2	3/2	U	U	U	U	2/1	2/1	2/2	3/3	2/1	2/2
58	Worm	11	M		M1	3/2	5/4	2/1	4/4	5/4	2/1	1/0	1/0	3/2	4/3	4/4
59	Worm	11	M		M1	U	3/2	U	U	U	4/3	3/2	2/2	3/2	4/3	D

60	Worm	11	M		M1	5/4	3/3	6/5	7/6	U	4/3	8/7	4/3	6/5	5/4	4/4
61	Worm	11	M		M1	2/1	4/3	3/3	3/3	2/1	U	1/0	2/1	U	U	U
71	Eust	11	M	15+	M1	1/0	U	1/0	2/1	2/1	3/2	4/3	4/4	5/5	6/6	5/5
72	Eust	10	M	11+	M1	5/5	5/5	4/3	U	U	6/5	6/6	7/6	8/7	8/8	9/8
82	Eust	11	M		M1	U	U	U	U	U	U	2/1	2/1	U	U	U
83	Eust	11	M		M1	1/0	2/1	1/1	1/0	1/0	U	1/0	2/1	1/1	1/1	1/1
85	Eust	10	M		M1	U	U	U	U	U	U	U	U	U	7/6	U
87	Eust	11	M		M1	1/0	2/1	1/0	1/0	1/1	U	2/1	1/1	1/1	2/2	1/1
88	Eust	10	M		M1	6/5	2/1	2/1	7/6	6/5	3/2	8/7	7/6	U	5/5	U
89	Eust	11	M	9	M1	7/6	U	U	10/9	7/6	8/7	6/5	7/7	11/11	U	11/10
90	Eust	11	M	9	M2	10/9	U	U	12/11	11/11	13/12	8/7	7/6	U	U	U
91	Eust	11	M		M1	U	U	U	U	U	U	U	U	11/10	9/9	12/11
99	Eust	10	F		M1	3/2	3/3	2/1	4/3	1/0	U	2/1	3/2	U	U	U
100	Eust	10	F		M1	D	D	7/6	5/4	4/3	6/5	D	D	8/7	3/3	7/6
103	Eust	11	M		M1	6/5	3/2	4/3	7/6	8/7	3/2	5/4	4/3	9/8	9/9	7/6
104	Eust	10	M		M1	3/2	5/4	U	U	6/6	6/5	5/4	4/4	U	U	4/4
105	Eust	12	M		M1	9/8	6/5	2/1	2/1	3/2	3/2	10/9	9/8	D	4/4	D
108	Eust	11	M	8-9	M1	8/7	7/6	5/4	8/7	6/5	4/3	7/6	5/4	6/5	8/8	5/5
109	Eust	11	M		M1	U	U	U	U	U	U	U	U	7/6	8/7	U
110	Eust	11	M	7-8	M1	U	U	6/5	5/4	U	U	8/7	7/6	U	7/7	U
112	Eust	10	M		M1	5/4	3/2	4/3	4/4	6/5	3/2	7/6	8/7	9/9	10/9	9/8
115	Eust	10	M	7-8	M1	U	U	11/10	11/11	U	U	9/8	14/13	12/12	9/9	U
116	Bal	12	U		M1	4/3	3/3	U	U	3/3	U	5/4	U	U	U	6/5
118	Bal	12	U		M1	3/3	2/2	2/1	U	D	1/0	3/3	5/4	U	U	U
119	Bal	12	U		M1	3/2	U	U	3/2	3/2	1/0	2/1	3/2	U	U	U
120	Bal	12	U		M1	1/0	U	U	U	2/1	2/1	2/1	3/3	U	U	U
122	Bal	12	U	2-3	M1	3/5	2/1	U	U	U	U	1/1	U	U	U	U
123	Bal	12	U		M1	1/1	U	2/2	2/2	2/1	1/0	2/2	4/4	U	U	U
124	Bal	12	U	4	M1	2/3	2/2	1/0	2/2	U	4/4	1/1	4/4	U	U	U
127	Str	8	M		M1	1/1	U	2/2	3/4	2/2	U	3/3	2/3	U	U	U
129	Str	8	M		M1	1/1	U	U	U	2/2	2/2	U	U	U	U	U
130	Str	8	M		M1	4/3	4/3	U	U	U	U	D	U	U	U	U
131	Str	8	M		M1	6/6	U	U	U	5/5	5/5	4/6	U	U	U	U
132	BAr	12	M	6-8	M1	4/3	2/1	6/5	7/6	3/2	2/1	7/6	9/8	U	3/3	U
135	CM	8	M	2	M1	2/1	2/1	1/0	U	U	2/1	2/2	3/2	2/2	2/2	3/2
136	CM	8	M		M1	3/2	U	U	2/2	2/1	1/0	3/2	2/2	U	U	U
141	High	10	M		M1	2/1	3/2	5/4	3/2	4/3	3/2	U	U	3/3	5/5	5/4
142	High	12	F		M1	U	U	U	U	U	U	1/0	1/0	U	U	U
143	High	12	F		M1	4/3	5/4	3/2	6/5	6/5	4/3	4/3	3/2	6/6	5/5	6/6
144	High	10	F		M1	3/2	2/1	5/4	2/2	4/3	4/3	3/3	3/2	D	D	D
145	High	10	M		M1	4/3	2/1	4/4	3/2	3/2	4/3	5/4	5/4	U	3/2	U
146	High	9	M	2	M1	1/0	2/1	2/1	1/0	1/1	U	U	1/0	2/2	3/2	2/1
147	High	9	M		M1	5/4	6/5	6/5	3/2	4/3	7/6	6/5	6/5	U	5/5	U
149	High	12	F		M1	4/3	6/5	U	U	8/7	7/6	U	8/7	6/6	5/5	U
152	Eust	10	M		M1	4/3	7/6	U	U	U	13/12	8/7	7/7	U	8/7	8/8
154	High	9	M		M1	2/1	1/0	1/0	3/2	2/1	U	U	3/2	3/3	2/2	3/3

155	High	9	M		M1	U	U	U	1/0	U	U	1/0	1/0	U	U	U
157	BAr	8	F		M1	5/4	3/2	3/2	2/1	4/3	4/3	4/3	3/3	3/3	4/4	3/3
162	BAr	9	M		M1	5/4	6/5	U	U	U	7/6	4/3	5/4	5/5	6/6	U
163	BAr	9	M		M1	1/0	2/1	2/1	1/0	3/2	2/1	2/1	1/0	2/2	3/3	2/2
167	Str	10	M		M2	3/2	1/1	1/1	2/1	2/2	2/1	2/2	4/3	U	U	U
171	Str	10	M		M1	U	2/1	3/2	U	1/0	U	2/1	1/2	U	U	U
173	Aber	10	M		M1	U	U	U	5/3	U	U	U	U	10/9	7/5	U
174	Aber	10	M		M1	U	U	4/3	U	U	U	3/2	U	U	6/5	6/6
176	High	9	F		M1	4/3	3/2	5/4	U	4/3	1/0	2/1	2/1	4/4	5/5	4/3
177	High	9	M		M1	2/1	2/1	1/0	1/1	2/1	1/0	2/2	1/1	3/3	2/1	2/2
178	High	10	F		M1	U	U	11/10	6/5	7/7	5/4	8/7	6/5	9/9	U	U
184	Bal	12	U		M3	2/1	U	U	U	U	1/0	U	U	U	U	U
185	Bal	12	U		M2	2/2	1/1	2/2	U	U	U	U	U	D	U	D
186	Bal	12	U		M1	1/1	D	1/0	U	U	U	1/1	1/1	U	U	U
187	Bal	12	U		M1	1/0	1/1	2/1	U	3/3	U	1/1	2/1	U	U	U
501	High	12	M	1.7	M1	1/1	1/1	2/2	2/2	1/1	1/1	1/1	2/2	2/2	2/2	1/1
502	High	1	M	2.8	M1	1/2	1/1	2/2	1/1	4/4	5/5	2/2	1/0	2/1	1/0	1/1
503	High	12	F	3.7	M1	2/2	2/2	2/2	1/0	3/3	3/2	3/3	3/3	D	6/6	2/2
504	High	10	F	4.5	M1	2/2	1/1	1/0	2/2	1/1	1/1	2/2	2/2	1/1	2/1	1/1
505	High	6	U	5.1	M1	3/3	2/2	2/2	3/3	5/4	3/3	4/4	4/5	D	5/5	D
506	High	7	M	6.2	M1	1/0	1/0	1/0	5/5	1/0	1/0	3/3	3/4	2/2	4/4	4/4
507	High	4	F	6.11	M1	1/0	5/5	3/3	5/4	1/0	6/4	2/1	6/5	2/2	5/5	3/3
508	High	11	U	7.6	M1	1/0	3/3	D	D	3/3	4/5	1/0	7/8	D	4/4	D
509	High	9	M	8.4	M1	2/2	6/5	9/8	1/0	6/5	5/5	1/0	1/0	3/2	5/5	2/2
510	High	8	M	9.3	M1	5/5	7/7	7/7	1/0	6/5	7/7	1/0	2/2	2/2	6/6	6/5
511	High	10	F	10.5	M1	D	1/0	8/8	3/3	D	1/0	D	4/5	6/6	5/5	6/6
512	High	1	F	10.8	M1	D	3/2	4/4	4/4	D	1/0	D	4/5	D	4/4	4/4
513	High	1	F	13.8	M1	3/2	8/9	U	6/5	5/4	U	5/5	7/6	1/0	1/0	1/0
514	High	9	F	16.4	M1	5/5	2/1	11/12	2/2	9/9	D	7/8	D	1/0	8/8	D

Table 13: Thin Section Data

Notice that there are a relatively large number of locations at which the sections are damaged or otherwise unreadable: the proportion of slides which are readable at each of the eleven locations is given in Table 14 below:

Location	Readable (%)
A	83.3
B	71.7
C	68.3
D	65
E	70.8
F	70.8
G	77.5
H	80.8
X	41.7
Y	59.2
Z	41.7

Table 14: Proportion of slides readable at each location

Observe the similarity between each symmetric pair of locations: A and H, B and G, X and Z, C and F, and D and E. The cellular cementum at the pad and apices (locations X, Y, and Z) is much more likely to be unreadable than the acellular cementum found elsewhere, with the pad being marginally better than the apices: locations A and H are most likely to provide clear and undamaged increments.

The remainder of this appendix provides analyses, first, of the known-aged sections, then of those of estimated age, and finally of the sample as a whole. It is clear that when the sample as a whole is being analysed, it is possible to study the discrepancies between layer counts at different locations around sections, but not to relate these to any age assessments. It is also important to bear in mind, in view of the very poor reliability of incremental analysis, that there is a large subjective element in the data being analysed.

The Known-age sample

Figures 71 to 81 are scatter plots of the number of bands observed, at each of the eleven standard locations, against the known age of the animals in question. Each plot includes a linear regression line through the data, together with its equation in the form $y = mx + c$. If it were the case that the number of bands gave a good approximation to age in years, then *m* would be close to 1, and *c* close to 0 in each case. In fact, *m* is substantially less than 1 at each of the 11 locations (the greatest value of *m* is 0.423, at location E), indicating that, in general, the number of observed bands increases by less than one for each year of the animal's life. The fact that almost all of the values of *m* are greater than zero indicates that there is some correlation between the number of bands observed and the age of the animal: this is unsurprising, given that the incremental structure is laid down over time. One might hope, in view of this, to be able to estimate the age of an animal from the number of bands and layers observed based on a relationship other than that of one band and one line being laid down annually. There are two reasons why the data does not support this hope. First, the values of *m* vary substantially between different locations around the root (from –0.001 to 0.423), indicating that the form of any such relationship would have to be very different at different locations. Second, the correlation coefficients R^2 (which are also shown in the plots) indicate the weakness of the correlation between the known age and the number of bands in each location. The correlation coefficients are greatest at locations A, E, G, and H (0.479, 0.519, 0.429, and 0.277 respectively), which are also the locations where the values of *m* are greatest: even at these locations, the correlation coefficients are low enough to indicate that there is no linear relationship between the number of bands and known age which is of any predictive value. The correlation coefficients at the pad and apical regions X, Y, and Z are very low (0.00003, 0.1682, and 0.2062 respectively). Indeed, the most cursory study of the plots shows, without any recourse to statistical analysis, the futility of attempting to obtain an accurate assessment of age on the basis of incremental analysis for this sample.

Figure 71: Number of bands at Location A against known age

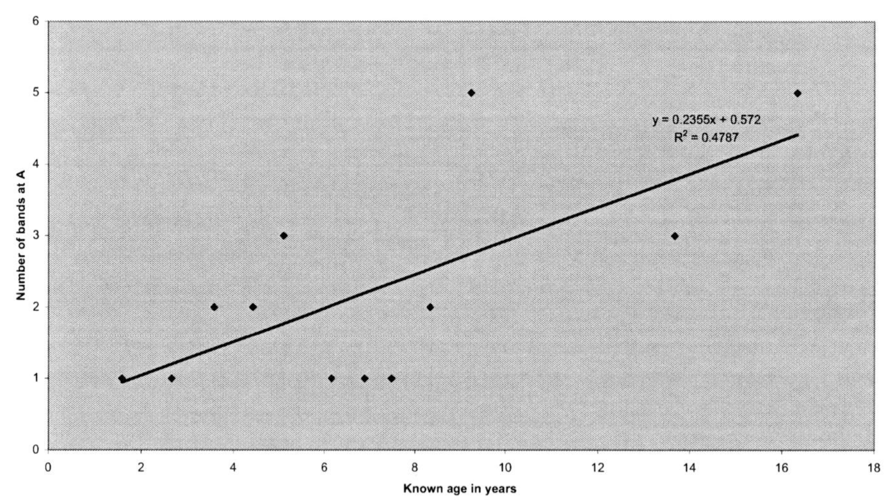

Figure 72: Number of bands at location B against known age

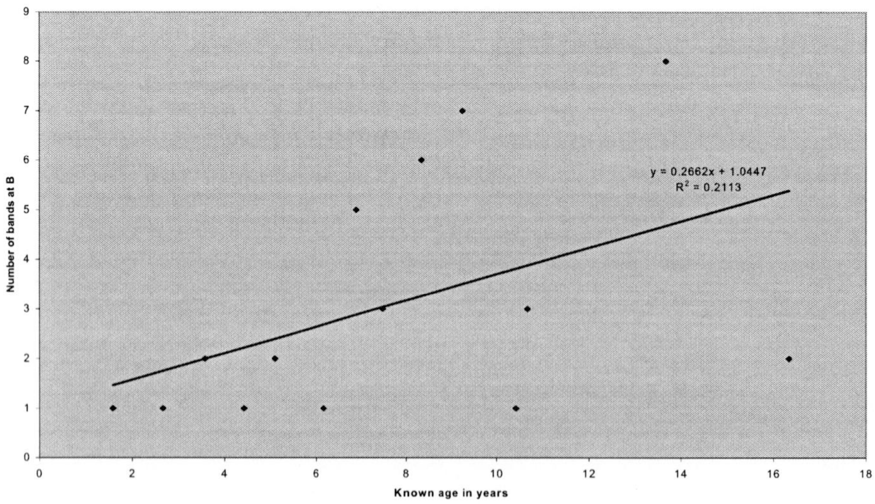

Figure 73: Number of bands at location C against known age

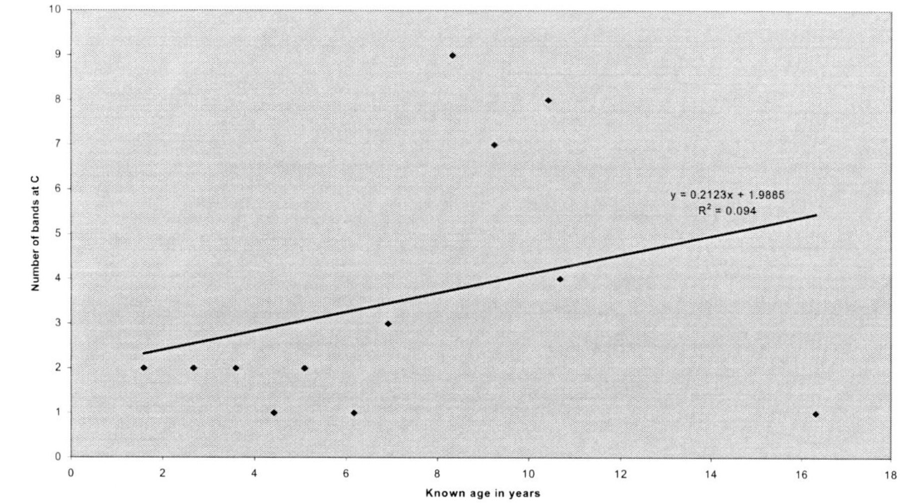

Figure 74: Number of bands at location D against known age

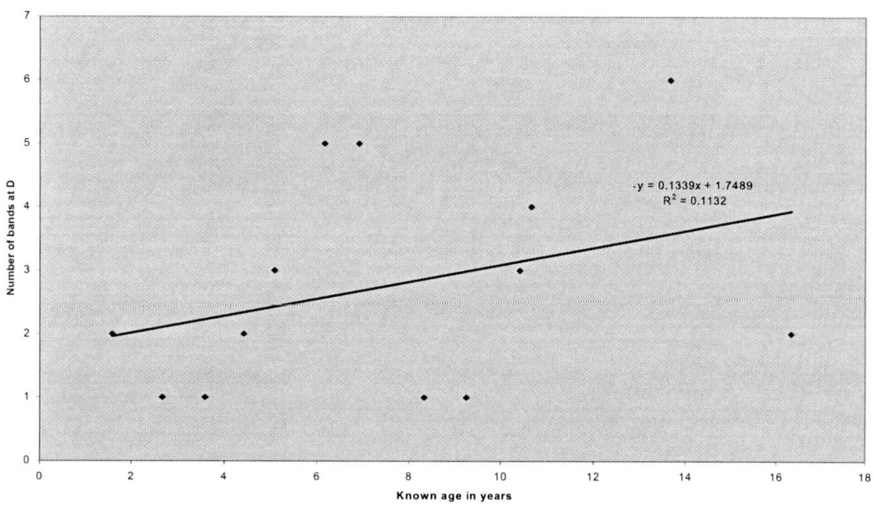

Figure 75: Number of bands at location E against known age

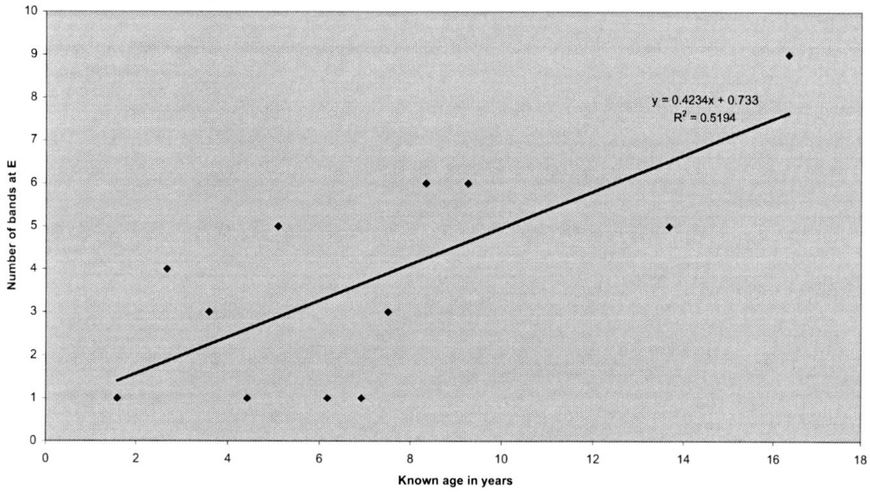

Figure 76: Number of bands at location F against known age

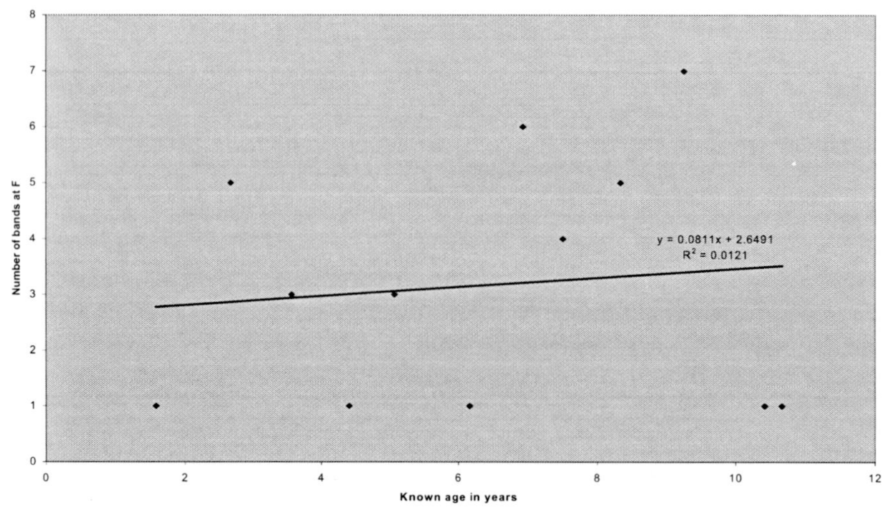

Figure 77: Number of bands at location G against known age

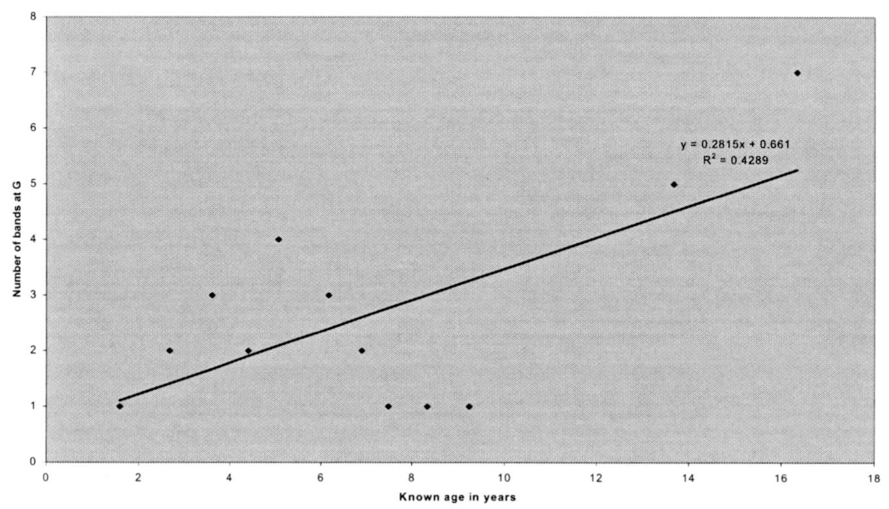

Figure 78: Number of bands at location H against known age

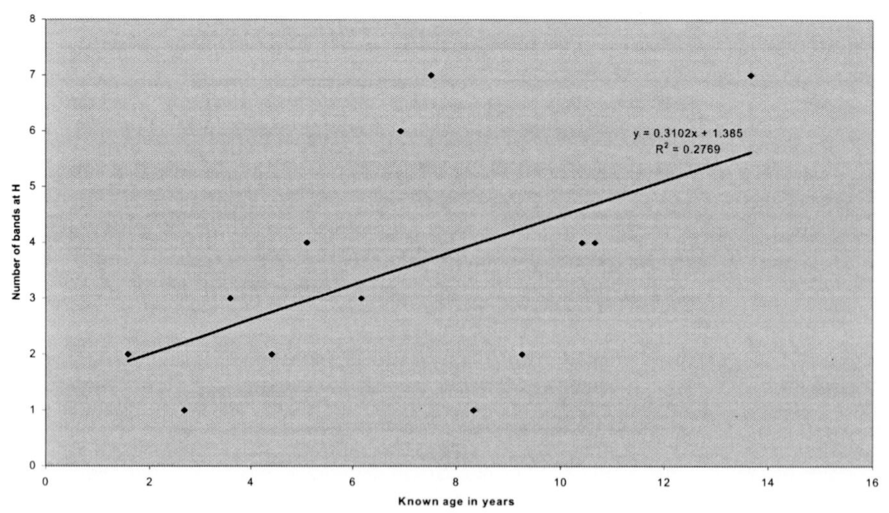

Figure 79: Number of bands at location X against known age

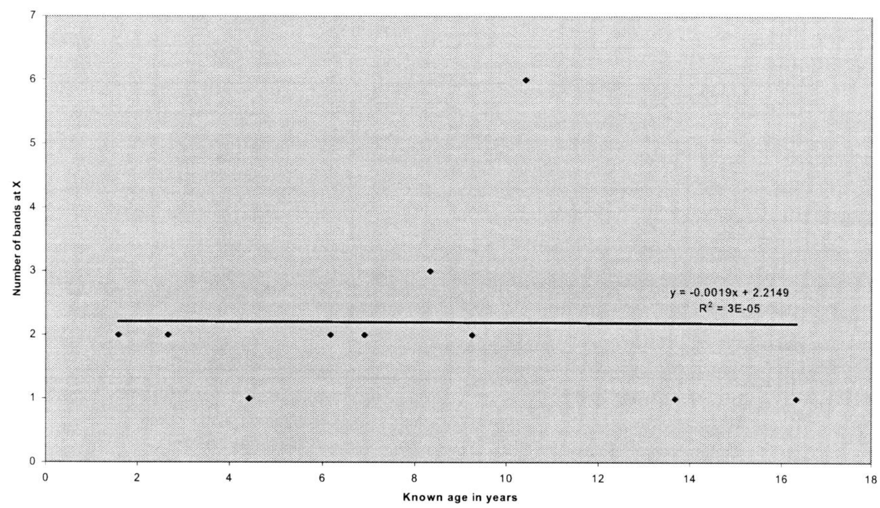

Figure 80: Number of bands at location Y against known age

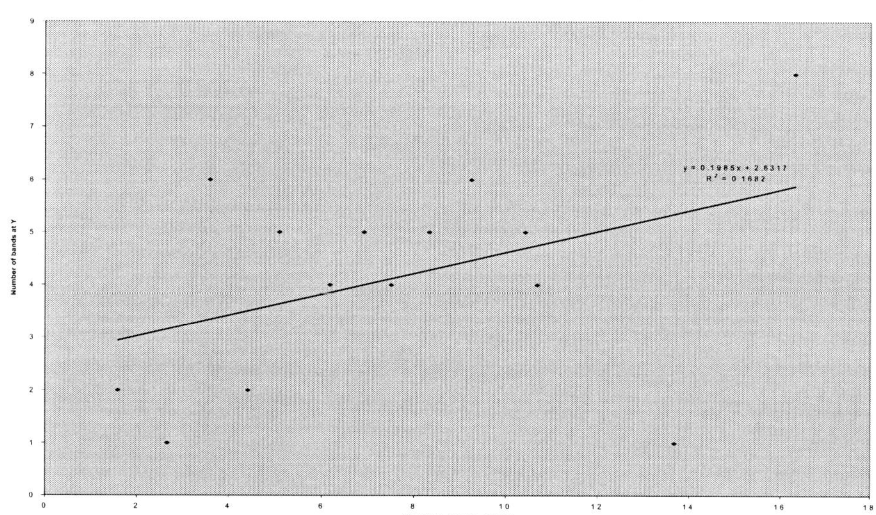

Figure 81: Number of bands at location Z against known age

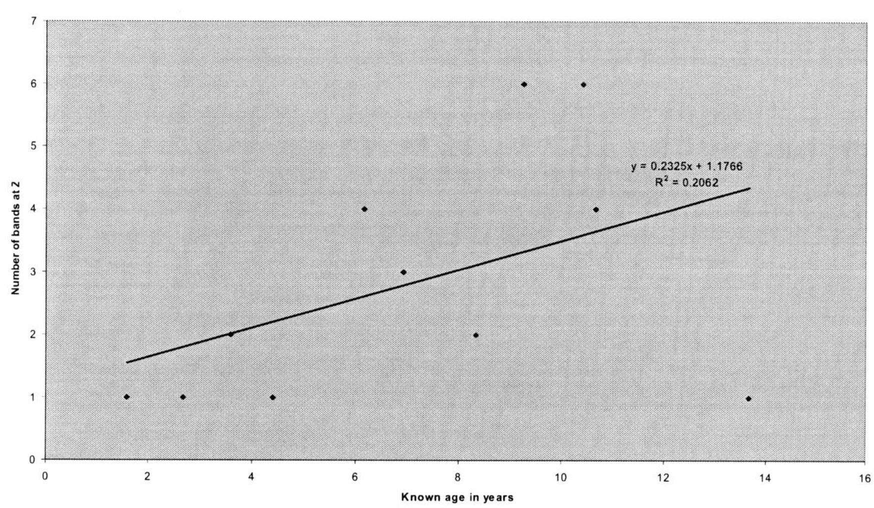

The p -values for these regressions (that is, the limiting levels of significance at which there is evidence to reject the hypothesis of no linear correlation) are as follows: location A, 0.012; location B, 0.098; location C, 0.332; location D, 0.261; location E, 0.008; location F, 0.734; location G, 0.021; location H, 0.064; location X, 0.987; location Y, 0.145; location Z, 0.161. Thus, for example, at a 5% level of significance, there is evidence to reject the hypothesis of no linear correlation at locations A, E, and G, and not at other locations; only at location E is there evidence to reject the hypothesis at a 1% level of significance. As has already been mentioned, it is unsurprising that there should be some correlation between the number of bands observed and the age of the animal, given that the incremental structure is laid down over time; on the other hand, it is also unsurprising that there may be no significant correlation at certain locations, especially since the measurements are taken from a sample of different animals, not from a single animal at different points during its life.

These plots and regression lines show that it is certainly not the case that the number of observed bands increases regularly at the rate of one each year for these sections. It is also possible to calculate the average and standard deviation of the discrepancies between the number of bands and the known age at each of the locations: the following results obtained are shown in Table 15. It can be seen that the average discrepancy is large at all eleven locations, especially when compared with the discrepancy for the scoring scheme as calculated in Chapter 6: recall that the average discrepancy for the scoring scheme was 17.21 months with a standard deviation of 18.9 months, these figures falling to 12.1 months and 11.3 months when only those animals yonger than 15 years were considered. The smallest average discrepancy in the table above, 3.6 years, translates to about 43 months. This study strongly suggests, therefore, that the scoring scheme provides a substantially more accurate method of ageing than does cementum incremental analysis.

Location	Average Discrepancy	Standard Deviation
A	4.88	3.50
B	4.54	3.76
C	3.80	4.09
D	4.92	4.04
E	3.60	2.79
F	3.60	3.08
G	4.46	3.44
H	3.47	2.91
X	5.86	4.79
Y	3.88	3.40
Z	4.24	3.38

Table 15: Average and standard deviation of discrepancy between known age and number of bands

Location	m	c	R^2	p-value	Mean discrepancy	Standard Deviation
A	0.086	2.170	0.0232	0.559	3.471	3.859
B	0.028	2.423	0.5468	0.005	2.615	2.895
C	0.075	1.933	0.0738	0.327	2.800	3.802
D	0.160	1.075	0.0189	0.612	3.500	3.864
E	0.018	3.136	0.0608	0.440	3.417	3.919
F	0.041	2.900	0.1927	0.089	3.375	3.302
G	0.152	3.059	0.5798	0.073	2.706	3.118
H	0.089	3.490	0.1845	0.075	2.778	2.922
X	-0.600	7.000	0.1920	0.238	3.667	3.571
Y	-0.077	5.833	0.4256	0.021	3.112	2.487
Z	-0.042	4.133	0.2580	0.134	3.400	3.169

Table 16: Analysis of the sample of estimated age

The Estimated-age Sample

An identical analysis was carried out for the sample of sections whose ages had been estimated by experienced stalkers. The results were very similar, but suffer from the confusion of uncertainty over the true age of the animal. A summary of the results, giving the equation $y = mx + c$ of the regression line, the correlation coefficient R^2, the p-value, and the average and standard deviation of the discrepancies between the number of bands and the estimated age at each location, is given in Table 16.

These results give no reason to doubt the conclusions of the analysis on the known-aged sample. One possible reason for the slightly improved (but still very large)

average discrepancies is that stalkers tend to underestimate the age of animals: since cementum incremental analysis also usually gives an underestimate of age, this would tend to decrease the discrepancy between the two methods of estimating age.

Analysis of the whole sample

Since the greater part of the sample was of neither known nor estimated age, it is meaningless to mimic the above analysis with the sample as a whole. Instead, a brief analysis was carried out of the variation between the number of bands observed at different locations around each of the 120 sections, by calculating for each slide the difference between the greatest and the smallest number of bands, taken over those locations where the section was readable. The frequency with which each possible such difference occurred in the sample is given in Table 17 below. Thus, for example, on 25 of the 120 sections there were three bands more at the location with the greatest number of bands then there were at the location with the smallest number of bands. The average such discrepancy is 3.25 bands, with a standard deviation of 2.163. On average, therefore, if a section is studied carefully around the whole of the tooth root, there will be an ambiguity of more than 3 years in the resulting age estimate. This emphasises the difficulty of making sensible, accurate, and reliable age estimates using cementum incremental analysis.

Discrepancy (bands)	Number of Sections
0	8
1	20
2	21
3	25
4	18
5	8
6	6
7	7
8	7

Table 17: Difference between largest and smallest numbers of bands at different locations

Bibliography

Adams, L and Watkins, S.G. 1967. Annuli in tooth cementum indicate age in California Grey squirrels. *Journal of Wildlife Management* **31(4)** 836-840.

Aiello, L.C. and Molleson, T. 1993. Are microscopic ageing techniques more accurate than macroscopic techniques?*Journal of Archaeological Science* **20** 689-704.

Aitken, R.J. 1975. Cementum layers and tooth wear as criteria for ageing Roe deer. *Journal of Zoology London* **175** 15-28.

Albright, D. 1989. Precision of seasonality determination in ringed seals *(Phoca hispida).* Paper presented at the 54th annual meeting of the society for American Archaeology, Atlanta.

Allen, S.H. 1974. Modified techniques for ageing Red fox using canine teeth. *Journal of Wildlife Management* **38(1)** 152-155.

Allen, S.H. and Kohn, S.C. 1976. Assignment of age classes in coyotes from canine cementum annuli. *Journal of Wildlife Management* **40:4** 796-797.

Allen, D.S. and Melfi, R.C. 1985. Improvements in techniques for ageing mammals by dental cementum annuli. *Proceedings Iowa Academy of Science* **92:3** 100-102.

Ambrose, S.H. 1990. Preparation and characterization of bone and tooth collegen for isotope analysis. *Journal of Archaeological Science* **17 4** 31-451.

Andersen, J.M., Byrd, B.F., Elson, M.D., Randall, H, McGuire, R.G., Mendoza, Staski, E, and White, J.P. 1981. The deer hunters: Star Carr reconsidered. *World Archaeology* **13/1** 30-46.

Armitage, P.L. 1975. The extraction and identification of opal phytoliths from the teeth of ungulates. *Journal of Archaeological Science* **2** 187-197.

Armitage, P.L. 1982. A system for ageing and sexing the horn cores of cattle from British post-medieval sites. *Ageing and sexing animal bones from archaeological sites BAR* **109** 37-54.

Armstrong, G. 1965. Tooth cementum of Bovidae with special reference to its use in age determination. *Science in Alaska* 29/30. Proceedings of the 16th Alaskan Science Conference, College, Alaska

Arthur, S.M. and Cross, R.A. 1992. Precision and utility of cementum annuli for estimating ages of Fishers. *Wildlife Society Bulletin* **20** 402-405.

Ascenzi, A.1969. Microscopy and Prehistoric bone. *Science in Archaeology* 526-538. Thames

Ashby, K.R. and Henry, B.A.M. 1979. Age criteria and life expectancy of Roe deer *(capreolus capreolus)* in the coniferous forest in North-Eastern England. *Journal of Zoology* **189(2)** 208-220.

Baales, M. and Street, M. 1996. Hunter-gatherer behaviour in a changing late glacial landscape: Allerod Archaeology in the central Rhineland, Germany. *Journal of Anthropological Research* **52** 281-316.

Banfield, A.W.F. 1960. The use of Caribou antler pedicles for age determination. *Journal of Wildlife Management* **24** 99-102.

Bang, G. and Ramn, E. 1970. Determination of age in humans from root dentine transparency. *Acta Odontologica Scandinavica* **28** 3-35.

Barth, E.K. 1983. Trapping Reindeer in South Norway. *Antiquity* **57** 109-115.

Bartos, L., Malik, V., Hyanek, J., Vavrunek, J., and Bytesnik, M. 1984. Relationship between rutting behaviour and non-annual incisor dentine layers of male Sika deer: A hypothesis. *Acta Theriol* **29** 431-435.

Baxter Brown, M. 1985. *Richmond Park - The history of a Royal deer park.* Robert Hale London

Baxter-Brown, M. 1990. Red deer twins:a note. *Journal of the British Deer Society* **8:1**.

Beasley, M.J. 1987. A preliminary report on incremental banding as an indicator of seasonality in mammal teeth from Gough's Cave, Cheddar, Somerset. *Proceedings of the University of Bristol Spelaeological Society* **18:1** 116-128.

Beasley, M.J., Brown, W.A.B. and Legge, A.J. 1992. Incremental banding in dental cementum: methods of preparation for teeth from archaeological sites and for modern comparative specimens. *International Journal of Osteoarchaeology* **2** 37-50.

Beeley, J.G. and Lunt, D.A. 1980. The nature of the biochemical changes in softened dentine from archaeological sites. *Journal of Archaeological Science* **7** 371-7.

Bell, L.S., Boyde, A. and Jones, S.J. 1991. Diagenetic alteration in teeth in situ illustrated by backscattered electron imaging. *Scanning* **13** 173-183.

Bell, L.S. 1990. Palaeopathology and diagenesis:An SEM evaluation of structural changes using backscattered electron imaging. *Journal of Archaeological Science* **17** 85-102.

Bellasis, H.R. 1991. The future for Red deer on Exmoor and the Quantocks. *Journal of the British Deer Society* 8:5.

Bender, B. 1978. Gatherer - hunter to farmer: a social perspective. *World Archaeology* **10** 204-222.

Berkovitz, B.K.B., Holland, G.R. and Moxham, B.J. 1995. *A colour atlas and text of oral anatomy, histology and embryology.* Second edition. Mosby-Wolfe, an imprint of Times Mirror International Publishers Limited.

Berzin, A.A. 1961. Materialy po razvitiyu zubov I opredeleniya vozrasta kashalota. (Materials on the development of teeth and age determination of the Sperm whale (*Physeter catodon). Trudy soveshchaniy ikhtiologicheskoi komissii.* **Issue 2**

Beynon, A.D. 1987. Replication technique for studying microstructure in fossil enamel. *Scanning Microscopy* **1:2** 663-669.

Bhaskar S.N. 1980. *Oral histology and embryology.*

Birgesson, B.and Ekvall, K. 1994. Suckling time and fawn growth in Fallow *deer (Dama dama). Journal of Zoology, London* **232** 641-650.

Blair, R.M. 1967. Deer forage in a loboly pine plantation. *Journal of Wildlife Management* **31(3)** 432-437.

Blair, R.M. and Brunett, L.E. 1980. Seasonal browse selection by deer in Southern Pine hardwood habitat. *Journal of Wildlife Management* **44(1)** 79-88.

Blankenhorn, H.J., Buchli, C. and Voser, P. 1978. Migration and seasonal distribution of Red deer *(Cervus elaphus)* in the Swiss National Park and its surroundings. *Rev-Suisse-Zool* **85:4** 779-789.

Bloom, W. and Fawcett, D.W. 1962. *A text book of histology 8th edition* 720. WB Saunders Co. Philadelphia

Bolus, M. and Street, M. 1996. Hunter-gatherer behaviour in a changing late glacial landscape: Allerod archaeology in the central Rhineland, Germany. *Journal of Anthropological Research* **52** 281-316.

Bosshardt, D.D. and Schroeder, H.E. 1996. Cementogenesis reviewed: a comparison between human premolars and rodent molars. *The Anatomical record.* **245** 267-292.

Bosshardt, D.D. and Selvig, K.A. 1997. Dental cementum: the dynamic tissue covering of the root. *Periodontology 2000.* **13** 41-75

Bothma, J., Teer, J.G. and Gates, C.E. 1972. Growth and age determination of the Cottontail in South Texas. *Journal of Wildlife Management* **36** 1209-1221.

Bourque, B.J., Morris, K. and Spiess, A. 1978. Determining the season of death of mammal teeth from archaeological sites: a new sectioning technique. *Science* **199** 530-1.

Bourque, B.J. 1975. Comments on the late Archaic populations of central Mains; the view from the Turner Farm. *Arctic Anthropology* **12** 35-45.

Bow, J.M. and Purday, C. 1966. A method of preparing Sperm whale teeth for age determination. *Nature* **210** 437-438.

Bowen, J. 1988. Seasonality: An agricultural construct. *Documentary archaeology in the New World.* Cambridge University Press

Boyde, A. 1987. Developmental interpretations of dental microstructure. Paper presented at the conference: Primate Life History and Evolution, Cabo san Lucas,Baja, Mexico,October, 1987

Boyde, A. 1971. Comparative histology of mammalian teeth. *Dental morphology and evolution* 81-94. Chicago University Press

Boyde, A. 1965. The structure of developing mammalian dental enamel. *Tooth enamel, International symposium on the composition, properties and fundamental structure of tooth enamel* 163-7. Bristol Wright

Boyde, A. 1963. Estimation of age at death of young human skeletal remains from incremental lines in the dental enamel. Third International meeting in Forensic Immunology, Medcine.(London 16-24April 1963)

Boyde, A., Petran, M. and Hadravsky, M. 1982. Tandem scanning reflected light microscopy of internal features in whole bone and tooth samples. *Journal of Microscopy* **132** 1-7.

Boyde, A. and Jones, S. 1972. Scanning Electron Microscopic studies of the formation of mineralised tissues. *Developmental aspects of oral biology* 234-274. New York Academic Press

Boyle, K.V. 1994. La madeleine (Tursac, Dordogne) une etude paleoeconomique du paleolithique superieur. *Paleo* **6** 55-77.

Bradford, E.W. 1967. Microanatomy and histochemistry of dentine. *Structural and chemical organization of teeth* 3-32. New York Academic Press

Bradley, J.A., Secord, D. and Prins, L. 1981. Age Determination in the Arctic fox *(Alopex lagopus). Canadian Journal of Zoology* **59(10)** 1976-1979.

Brewer, D. 1989. Chronologies and palaeoenvironments:incremental growth structures of the Nile Perch *(Lates niloticus)*. Paper presented at 54th annual meeting of Society for American Archaeology, Atlanta

Brewer, D. 1987. Seasonality in the prehistoric Faijum based on the incremental growth structures of the Nile catfish *(Pisces claris). Journal of Archaeological Science* **14** 459-472.

Brokx, P.A. 1972. Age determination of Venezuelan White-tailed deer. *Journal of Wildlife Management* **36(4)** 1060-1067.

Brothwell, D. 1963. *Dental anthropology* Pergaman, New York.

Brown, W.A.B. and Chapman, N.G. 1991. The dentition of Red deer *(Cervus elaphus):* a scoring scheme to assess age from wear of the permanent molariform teeth. *Journal of Zoology London* **224** 519-536.

Brown, W.A.B. and Chapman, N.G. 1991. Age assessment of Fallow deer *(Dama dama):* from a scoring scheme based on radiographs of developing permanent molariform teeth. *Journal of Zoology London* **224** 367-379.

Brown, W.A.B. and Chapman, N.G. 1990. The dentition of Fallow deer *(Dama dama):* a scoring system to assess age from the wear of the permanent molariform teeth. *Journal of Zoology London* **221** 659-682.

Brown, W.A.B., Christofferson, P.V., Massler, M. and Weiss, M.B. 1960. Postnatal tooth development in cattle. *American Journal of Veterinary Research* **21:80** 7 -34.

Brown, W.A.B. 1982. Resorption of permanent teeth. *British Journal of Orthodontics* **9** 212-220.

Brown, W.A.B. 1985. Identification of human teeth. *Bulletin* **21/22** 1-30.

Bull, G. and Payne, S. 1982. Tooth eruption and epiphyseal fusion in pigs and wild boar. *Ageing and sexing animal bones from archaeological sites BAR* **109** 55-71.

Bullock, D. and Rackham, J. 1982. Epiphysial fusion and tooth eruption of feral goats from Moffatdale, Dumfries and Galloway, Scotland. *Ageing and Sexing Animal bones fromAarchaeological sites BAR* **109** 73-80.

Burke, A. 1993. Applied skeletochronology: the horse as human prey during the Pleriglacial in South Western France. *Archaeological Papers of American Anthropological Association.* **4** 145-150.

Burke, A.M. 1993. Observation of incremental growth structures in dental cementum using the scanning electron microscope. *Archaeozoologia* **5:2** 41-54.

Burke, A. 1992. Prey Movements and settlement patterns during the Upper Palaeolithic in Southwestern France. PhD thesis, New York University.University Microfilms,Ann Arbor,Michigan

Burke, A. and Castanet, J. 1995. Histological observations of cementum growth in horse teeth and their application to archaeology. *Journal of Archaeological Science* **22** 479-493.

Butler, P.M. & Joysey, K.A.(eds) 1978. *Development, function and evolution of teeth.* London : Academic Press.

Carlson, S. and Carter, J.1990. Vertebrate Dental structures. *Skeletal biomineralization: patterns, processes and evolutionary trends.* 1 531-556. Van Nostrand Reinhold.NY

Carrick, R. and Ingham, S.E. 1962. Studies on the Southern Elephant seal *(Mirounga leonina)* L.II : Canine tooth structure in relation to function and age determination. *Wildlife Research* **7:2** 102-118.

Carter, R.J. 1997. Age estimation of the Roe deer *(Capreolus capreolus)* mandibles from the Mesolithic site of Star Carr, Yorkshire, based on radiographs of mandibular tooth development. *Journal of Zoology London* **241** 495-502.

Carter, R.J. 1998. Reassessment of seasonality at the early Mesolithic site of Star Carr, Yorkshire, based on radiographs of mandibular tooth development in Roe deer *(Cervus elaphus). Journal of Archaeological Science* **25** 851-856

Castanet, J. 1981. Nouvelles donnees sur les lignes cimentantes de l'os. *Archives Bibliogiques* **92** 1-24.

Casteel, R.W. 1976. Incremental growth zones in mammals and their archaeological value. *Papers of the Krober Anthropological Society (Berkeley)* **47** 1-27.

Caulfield, S. 1978. Star Carr- an alternative view. *Irish Archaeological Research Forum* **5** 15-22.

Chaplin, R.E. and White, R.W.G. 1969. The use of tooth eruption and wear, body weight and antler characteristics in the age estimation of male wild and park Fallow deer *(Dama dama). Journal of Zoology* **157** 125-32.

Chapman, N., Claydon, K., Claydon, M., Forde, P.G. and Harris, S. 1993. Sympatic populations of Munjack *(Muntiacus reevesi)* and Roe deer *(Capreolus capreolus)*: a comparative analysis of their ranging behaviour, social organisation and activity. *Journal of Zoology London* **229** 623-640.

Chapman, N.G. and Furlong, M. 1997. Reproductive strategies and the influence of date of birth on growth and sexual development of an a seasonally-breeding ungulate:

Reeve's Muntjack *(Muntiacus reevesi). Journal of Zoology London* **241** 551-570.

Chapman, D.I. and Chapman, N.G. 1970. Development of the teeth and mandibles of Fallow deer *(Dama dama). Acta theriologica* **15** 111-131.

Chapman, D.I. and Chapman, N.G.1997. *Fallow Deer.*Coch-Y-Bonddu Books.

Charles, B.K., Condon, K. and Buikstra, J.E. 1986. Cementun annulation and age determination in Homo sapiens I: tooth variability and observer error. *American Journal of Physical anthropology* **71** 311-320.

Chrisholm, B.S., Nelson, D.E. and Schwarcz, H.P.1983. Carbon isotope measurement techniques for bone collagen: notes for the archaeologists. *Journal of Archaeological Science* **10** 355-360.

Clark, J.G.D. 1972. *Star Carr: a case study in Bioarchaeology*. Addison-Wesley

Clark, J.G.D. 1954. *Excavations at Starr Carr an Early Mesolithic Site at Seamer near Scarborough, Yorkshire.* Cambridge University Press

Clark, J.G.D. 1950. A preliminary report on excavations at Star Carr, Seamer, Scarborough, Yorkshire (second season 1950). *Proceedings of the Prehistoric Society* **XVI** 109-128.

Clark, J.G.D. 1949. A preliminary report on excavations at Star Carr, Seamer, Scarborough, Yorkshire, 1949. *Proceedings of the Prehistoric Society* **XV** 52-69.

Clark, J.G.D. 1936. *The Mesolithic settlement of Northern Europe. A study of the food-gathering peoples of Northern Europe during the post-glacial period.* Cambridge University Press

Clawson, R.G. and Causey, M.K. 1995. Dental casts for White-tailed deer age estimation. *Wildlife Society Bulletin* **23(1)** 92-94.

Clevedon Brown, J. 1979. Techniques in mammalogy. Microscopical examination:histological methods. *Mammal Review* **9(3)**

Clevedon Brown, J. and Hilton, A.J. 1979. Techniques in mammalogy. Microscopical examination:histological technique. *Mammal Review* **9(2)**

Clutton-Brock, T. 1983. Why study large animals? *New Scientist* **100** 193-9.

Clutton-Brock, T.H. and Albon, S.D. 1989. *Red deer in the Highlands.* BSP Professional Books

Clutton-Brock, T.H. and Albon, S.H. 1983. Climatic variation and body weight of Red deer. *Journal of Wildlife Management* **47:4** 1197-1201.

Clutton-Brock, T.H. and Guinness, F.E. 1982. *Red deer behaviour and ecology of two sexes.* Edinburgh University Press

Clutton-Brock, T.H. and Lonergon, M.E. 1994. Culling regimes and sex ratio biases in Highland Red deer. *Journal of Applied Ecology* **31:3** 521-527.

Clutton-Brock, J. and Noe-Nygaard, N. 1990. New Osteological and C-isotope evidence on Mesolithic dogs: Companions to hunters and fishers at Star Carr, Seamer Carr and Kongemose. *Journal of Archaeological Science* **17** 643-653.

Coe, R.J., Downing, R.L. and McGinnes, B.S. 1980. Sex and age bias in hunter-killed White tailed deer. *Journal of Wildlife Management* **44(1)** 245-249.

Condon, K., Charles, D.K., Cheverud, J.M. and Buikstra, J.E. 1986. Cementum annulation and age determination in Homo sapiens II: estimates and accuracy. *American Journal of Physical Anthropology* **71** 321-330.

Cook, R.L. and Hart, R.V. 1979. Ages assigned known-age Texas White-tailed deer: Tooth wear versus cementum analysis. *Proceedings Annual Conference South East Association Fish & Wildlife Agencies* **33** 195-201.

Corner, E.J.H. 1950. Report on Fungus - brackets from Star Carr, Seamer. *Proceedings of the Prehistoric Society* **16** 123-124.

Coutts, P. and Higham, C. 1971. The seasonal factor in prehistoric New Zealand. *World Archaeology* **2:3** 266-277.

Coy, J.P. and Jones, R.T. 1982. Absolute ageing in cattle from tooth sections and its relevance to archaeology. Ageing and sexing animal bones from archaeological sites *BAR British series* **109** 127-140.

Craighead, J.J., Craighead, F.C. and McCutchen, H.E. 1970. Age determination of Grizzly bears from fourth premolar sections. *Journal of Wildlife Management* **34:2** 353-364.

Cross, J.R., Hitchcock R.K. 1989. Expanding the scope of seasonality research in archaeology. Philadelphia PA: MASCA Research papers in Science & Archaeology **(vol 5)** *Coping with seasonal constraints* 55-63.

Crowe, D.M. 1972. The presence of annuli in Bobcat tooth cementum layers. *Journal of Wildlife Management.* **36 (4)** 1330-32

Crowe, D.M. and Strickland, N.D. 1975. Dental annulations in the American badger. *Journal of Mammals* **56** 269-272.

Cruwys, E. & Foley, R. 1986. Cementum deposition among tropical African ungulates:implications for

Palaeolithic studies. Teeth and Anthropology. *BAR International Series* **291** 83-99

Dapson, R.W. 1980. Guidelines for statistical usage in age-estimation techniques. *Journal of Wildlife Management* **44:3** 541-548.

Darling, F.F. 1937. *A herd of Red deer: a study in animal behaviour.* Edinburgh University Press.

Davis, W.L. 1986. The archaeology of animals. *Oral Histology.* Edinburgh University Press.

Davis, S.J.M. 1983. The age profiles of gazelles predated by ancient man in Israel:possible evidence for a shift from seasonality to sedentism in the Natufian. *Paleorient* **9** 55-62.

Davis, S.J.M. 1987. *Archaeology of Animals.* Batsford Ltd London

Day, S.P. 1993. Preliminary results of high -resolution Palaeoecological analysis at Star Carr Yorkshire. *Cambridge Archaeological Journal* **3:1** 129-133.

Day, S.P. and Mellars, P.A. 1994. 'Absolute' dating of Mesolithic human activity at Star Carr, Yorkshire: new Palaeoecological studies and identification of the 9600BP Radiocarbon 'Plateau'. *Proceedings of the Prehistoric Society* **60** 417-422.

Day, S.P. 1996. Devensian Late glacial and early Flandrian environmental history of the Vale of Pickering, Yorkshire, England. *Journal of Quaternary Science* **11** 9-24.

Day, S.P. 1996. Dogs, deer and diet at Star Carr: a reconsideration of c-isotope evidence from early Mesolithic dog remains form the Vale of Pickering, Yorkshire, England. *Journal of Archaeological Science* **23** 783-787.

Delap, P. 1988. Rhum goings on. *Journal of the British Deer Society* **7:6**

Demirjian, A., Goldstein, H. and Tanner, J.M. 1973. A new system of dental age assessment. *Human Biology* **45** 211-227.

Deniz, E. and Payne, S. 1982. Eruption and wear in the mandibular dentition as a guide to ageing Turkish Angora goats. . Ageing and sexing animal bones from archaeological sites *British Archaeological Reports British Series* **109** 155-205.

Deutsch, D., El-Attar, I., Robinson, C. and Weatherall, J.A. 1979. Rate and timing of enamel development in the deciduous bovine incisor. *Archives of Oral Biology* **24** 407-13.

Dills, G.G. 1970. Effects of prescribed burning on deer browse. *Journal of Wildlife Management* **34:3** 540-5.

Doberenze, A.R. and Wyckoff, W.G. 1967. The microstructure of fossil teeth. *Journal of Ultrastructure Research* **18** 166-75.

Douglas, M. 1970. Dental cement layers as criteria of age of deer in New Zealand with the emphasis on Red deer *(Cervus elaphus). New Zealand Journal of Science* **13** 352-358.

Douglas, K.C., Condon, K., Chevervol, J.M. and Bruikstra, J.E. 1989. Estimating age at death from growth layer groups in cementum. *Age markers in the human skeleton* 277-301.

Douglas, K., Condon, C.K., Cheverud, J.M. and Buikstra, J.E. 1986. Cementum annulation and age determination in Homo sapiens 1. Tooth variability and observer error. *American Journal of Physical Anthropology* **71** 311-320.

Dudley, T. 1996. Deer ancient and modern. *Journal of the British Deer Society* **10:2** 82-85.

Dumont, J.V. 1983. An interim report of the Star Carr microwear study. *Oxford Journal of Archaeology* **2(2)** 127-145.

Eidermann, N. 1932. Alterserscheinungen am gebiss des Rothirsches *(Cervus elaphus.L). Mitt.Forstw.Fortwiss* **3** 291-341.

Edwards, K.J. and Hirons, K.B. 1984. Cereal pollen grains in pre elm decline deposits: Implications for the earliest agriculture in Britain and Ireland. *Journal of Archaeological Science* **11** 71-80.

Elder, W.H. 1965. Primeval deer hunting pressures revealed by remains from American Indian middens. *Journal of Wildlife Management* **29** 366-370.

Erickson, J.A., Anderson, A.E., Medin, D.E. and Bowden, P.C. 1970. Estimating ages of Mule deer- an evaluation of technique accuracy. *Journal of Wildlife Management* **34** 523-531.

Erickson, J.A. and Seliger, W.G. 1969. Efficient sectioning of incisors for estimating ages of Mule deer. *Journal of Wildlife Management* **33** 384-388.

Fancy, S.G. 1980. Preparation of mammalia teeth for age determination by cementum layers:a review. *Wildlife Society Bulletin* **8** 242-8.

Fisher, H.D. and McKenzie, B.A. 1954. Rapid preparation of tooth sections for age determination. *Journal of Wildlife Management* **18** 537-7.

Fleiss, J.L. 1986. *The design and analysis of clinical experiments.* Wiley, New York.

Fogl, J.G. and Mosby, H.S. 1978. Ageing Grey squirrels by cementum annuli in razor-sectioned teeth. *Journal of Wildlife Management* **42** 444-8.

Foley, R. 1986. Cementum deposition among tropical African ungulates: Implications for Palaeological studies. Teeth and archaeology *BAR* **291**, 83-99.

Francillan-Vieillot, H., De Buffrenil, V., Castanet, J., Geraudie, J., Meunier, F.J., Sire, J.Y., Zylberberg, L. and De Ricqles, A. 1991. Microstructure and mineralization of vertebrate skeletal tissues. *Skeletal biomineralization: patterns, processes and evolutionary trends* 471-530. Van Nostrand NY

Fraser, F.C. and King, J.E. 1950. Second interim report on the animal remains from Star Carr, Seamer. *Proceedings of the Prehistoric Society* **16** 124-129.

Fraser, F.C. and King, J.E. 1949. The bone remains from Star Carr. *Proceedings of the Prehistoric Society* **15** 67-69.

Free, S. and Saver, P.R. 1966. Cementum layering in the canine tooth of a 28yr old captive Black bear. *New York Fish Game Journal* **13** 233-234.

Frison, G.C. and Wilson, M. 1976. *American Antiquity* **41** 28.

Frison, G.C. and Rehler, C.A. 1970. Age determination of Buffalo by teeth eruption and wear. *Plains Anthropologist* The Glenrock buffalo jump 48 **15(2.2)** 46-47.

Frost, H.M. 1958. Preparation of thin uncalcified bone sections by rapid manual method. *Stain Technology* **33(6)** 273-277.

Frylestam, B. and von Schantz, T. 1977. Age determination of European hares based on periostal growth lines. *Mammal Review* **7(3/4)** 151-4.

Furseth, R. 1970. A microradiographic and light microscope and electron microscope study of the cementum from deciduous teeth of pigs. *Actaodent Scandanavia* **28** 833-850.

Gabe, M. 1976. *Histological techniques* Paris & Berlin

Gantt, D.G. 1979. A method of interpreting enamel prism pattern. *Scanning Electron Microscopy* 491-496.

Gasaway, W.C., Harkness, D.B. and Rausch, R.A. 1978. Accuracy of Moose age determinations from incisor cementum layers. *Journal of Wildlife Management* **42** 558-63.

Gilbert. A.S. 1989. Microscopic bone structure in wild and domestic animals: a reappraisal. *Early Animal Domestication and its Cultural Context* 46-86 MASCA Research Papers in Science and Archaeology, Philadelphia.

Gilbert, BM. 1980. *Mammalian osteology* Laramie

Gilbert, BM. 1973. *Mammalian osteo-archaeology: North America.* Missouri Archaeological Society, Columbia

Gilbert, F.F. 1966. Ageing White-tailed deer by annuli in the cementum of the first incisor. *Journal of Wildlife Management* **30(1)** 200-2.

Gilbert, F.F. and Solt, S.L. 1970. Variability in ageing Maine White-tailed deer by tooth wear characteristics. *Journal of Wildlife Management*, **34** 532-5.

Glimcher, M.J. and Lefteiou, B. 1989. Soluble glycosylated phosphoprotiens of cementum. *Calcified Tissue International* **45** 165-172.

Goddard, H.N. and Reynolds, J.C. 1993. Age determination in Red fox (Vulpes vulpes) from cementum lines. *Game Conservancy Age Structure UK* 173-187.

Godwin, H. 1949. Preliminary reports on peat-stratigraphy and pollen analysis in the Flixton-Seamer area. *Proceedings of the Prehistoric Society* **15** 65-67.

Gordon, B.C. 1989. Archaeological tooth and bone seasonal increments: the need for standardised terms and techniques. *Archaeozoologia* **5:2** 9-16.

Gordon, B.C. 1988. Of Men and Reindeer herds in French Magdalenian Prehistory *BAR* **390** Oxford

Gordon, B.C. 1985. Seasonal indications of parallel band movements in Canadian Barrenland and French Magdalenian prehistory. Paper presented at the 84th annual meeting of the American Anthropological Association, Washington DC

Gordon, B.C. 1984. Selected bibliography of dental annular studies on various mammals. *Zooarchaeological Research News, Supplement Number Two.*

Gordon, B.C. 1982. Tooth Sectioning as an Archaeological Tool. *National Museum of Man, Archaeological Survey of Canadian Studies.* **14**

Gordon, B.C. 1991. Archaeological seasonality using incremental structures in teeth. An annotated bibliography. A special publication of *Zooarchaeological Research News.* New York.

Grant, A. 1982. The use of tooth wear as a guide to the age of domestic animals. *Ageing and sexing animal bones from archaeological sites BAR (British Series)* **109** 91-108.

Grau, G.A., Sanderson, G.C. and Rogers, J.P. 1970. Age determination of racoons. *Journal of Wildlife Management* **34:2** 364-372.

Grayson, D. 1984. *Quantitive zooarchaeology* Academic Press, New York

Grayson, D.K. 1979. On the quantification of vetebrate archaeofaunas. *Advances in archaeological method and theory* 199-237. Academic Press, New York.

Grayson, D.K. 1978. Minimum numbers and sample size in vertebrate faunal analysis. *American Antiquity* **43** 53-65.

Grayson, D.K. 1973. On the methodology of faunal analysis. *American Antiquity* **38** 432-439.

Green, J. and Barghi, N. 1989. Comparative study of three polishing agents on loss of cementum. *Journal of Dental Research* **68**

Greer, K. and Yeager, H. 1967. Sex and age indications from upper canine teeth of Elk (wapiti). *Journal of Wildlife Management* **31:3** 408-417.

Grevstad, H.J. and Selvig, K.A. 1985. Location and ultrastructure of the first cementum formed in rabbit incisors. *Journal of Dental Research* **93** 289-303.

Grigson, C. 1981. Fauna. *The environment of British prehistory.* 101-124. London: Duckworth.

Grimsdell, J.J.R. 1973. Age Determination of the African Buffalo, *(Syncerus caffer Sparrman) East African Wildlife Journal* **11** 31-53.

Grimstone, A.V. and Skaer, R.J. 1972. *A guidebook to microscopical methods*. Cambridge University Press

Grue, H. 1976. Non-seasonal incremental lines in tooth cementum of domestic *dogs (Canis familiaris,L)* of known age. *Danish Review of Game Biology* **10 (2)** 2-8.

Grue, H. and Jensen, B. 1979. Review of the formation of incremental lines in tooth cementum of terrestrial mammals. *Danish Review of Game Biology* **11(3)** 1-48.

Grue, H. and Jensen, B. 1976. Annual cementum structures in canine teeth in Arctic foxes *(Alopex lagopus L)* from Greenland and Denmark. *Danish Review of Game Biology* **10(3)**
3-12.

Grue, H. and Jensen, B. 1973. Annular structures in cannine tooth cementum in Red foxes *(Vulpes vulpes)* of known age. *Danish Review of Game Biology* **8(7)** 1-12.

Guinness, F.E., Gibson, R.M. and Clutton-Brock, T.H. 1978. Calving times of Red deer *(Cervus elephus)* on Rhum. *Journal of Zoology Proceedings London* **185** 105-114.

Gustafson, C.E. 1968. *Science* **49**

Habermehl, K.H. 1961. *Die alterbestimmung bei haustieren, pelztieren und beim jagdbarer, wildtieren* Hamburg & Berlin

Hackett, E., Guynn, J.C.D. and Jacobson, H.A. 1979. Differences in age structure of White-tailed deer in Mississippi produced by two ageing techniques. *Proceedings 0f the Annual Conference of the South East Association of Fish &Wildlife Agencies* **33** 25-29.

Hagg, U. and Matsson, L. 1985. Dental maturity as an indicator of chronological age: the accuracy and precision of three methods. *European Journal of Orthodontics* **7** 25-34.

Hall-Martin, A.J. 1976. Dentition and age-determination of the giraffe *(Giraffa Camelopardalis). Journal of Zoology London* **180** 263-289.

Hamilton, J. 1982. Re-examination of a sample of Iron Age sheep mandibles from Ashville Trading Estate, Abingdon, Oxfordshire. Ageing and sexing animal bones from archaeological sites *BAR* **109** 215-222.

Harris, S. 1978. Age determination in the Red fox *(Vulpes vulpes)* an evaluation of technique efficiency as applied to a sample of suburban foxes. *Journal of Zoology London* **184** 91-117.

Harris, R.A. and Duff, K.R. 1970. *Wild deer in Britain.* Taplinger Publishing Co.New York

Hartman, G. 1992. Age determination of live Beaver by dental X-Ray. *Wildlife Society Bulletin* **20(2)** 216-220.

Hawkins, R.E., Autry, D.C. and Klimstra, W.D. 1967. Comparison of methods used to capture White-tailed deer. *Journal of Wildlife Management* **31(3)** 460-464.

Hemming, J.E. 1969. Cemental deposition, tooth succession, and horn development as criteria of age in Dall sheep. *Journal of Wildlife Management* **33** 552-558.

Henderson Scott, J. and Barrington Bray Symo, N. 1982. *Introduction to dental anatomy*. Churchill Livingstone

Henry, B.A.M. 1978. Diet of Roe deer in an English conifer forest. *Journal of Wildlife Management* **42:4** 937-940.

Hewer, H.R. 1964. The determination of age, sexual maturity, longevity and a life table in the Grey seal *(Halichoerus grypus). Journal of Zoology Proceedings London* **142:4** 593-624.

Hewer, H.R. 1960. Age determination of seals. *Nature* **186** 959-960.

Higgs, E.S. and White, P.J. 1963. Autumn killing. *Antiquity* **148** 282-289.

Hillman-Smith, A.K.K., Owen-Smith, N., Anderson, J.L., Hall-Martin, A.J. and Selaldi J.P. 1986. Age estimation of the White rhinoceros *(Ceratotherium simum). Journal of Zoology London* **210** 355-79.

Hillson, S.W. 1992. Impression and replica methods for studying hypoplasia and perikymata on human tooth crown surfaces from archaeological sites. *International Journal of Osteoarchaeology* **2** 65-78.

Hillson, S.W. 1986. *Teeth*. Cambridge University Press.

Hillson, S. 1988. The scanning electron microscope and the study of ancient teeth. Scanning electron microscopy in archaeology *BAR International Series* **452** 249-260.

Hingston, F. *Deer parks and deer of Great Britain.*

Holmbäck, A.M., Porter, M., Downham, D.Y. and Lexell, J. 1999. Reliability of isokinetic ankle dorsiflexor strength measurements in young healthy men and women. *Scandinavian Journal of Rehabilitation Medicine.* In Press.

Hubbard, R.N.L. 1995. Fallow deer in prehistoric Greece, and the analogy between faunal spectra and pollen analysis. *Antiquity* **69** 527-38.

Hudson, D. 1992. Antler casting and regrowth in Red deer. *Journal of the British Deer Society* **8:8**

Humphries, D.W. 1992. The preparation of Thin Sections of rocks, minerals and ceramics. *Microscopy Handbooks* **24** Oxford University Press.

Illius, A.W. and Gordon, I.J. 1990. Variation in foraging behaviour in Red deer and the consequences for population demography. *Journal of Animal Ecology* **59(1)** 89-102.

Ismaul, O.S. and Weber, D.F. 1986. Scanning electron microscopy of casts of cellular cementum. *Journal of Dental Research* **65** 264.

Jacobi, R.M., Tallis, J.H. and Mellars P.A. 1976. The Southern Pennine Mesolithic and the ecological record. *Journal of Archaeological Science* **3** 307-320.

Jacobi, R.M. 1978. Northern England in the eighth millennium BC: an essay. *The early post glacial settlement of Northern Europe. An ecological perspective.* 295-332. London: Duckworth.

Jacobson, H.A. and Reiner, R.J. 1989. Estimating Age of White-tailed deer: Tooth wear versus cementum annuli. *Proceedings of the Annual Conference of the South East Association of Fish & Wildlife Agencies* **43** 286-291.

Jeffs, C. and Benstead, P. 1995. Roe Deer Preliminary Data Analysis.

Jensen, B., Nielsen, L.B. and Brunberg, L. 1968. Age determination in the Red fox *(Vulpes vulpes)* from canine tooth sections. *Danish Review of Game Biology* **5(6)** 3-15.

Johnson, R. 1987. A classification of Sharpey's fibres within the aveolar bone of the mouse:a high voltage electron microscope study. *The Anatomical Record* **217** 339-347.

Jones, S.J. 1987. The root surface: an illustrated review of some scanning electron microscope studies. *Scanning Microscopy* **1** 2003-18.

Jones, S.J. 1981. Dental tissues: cement *Dental Anatomy and Embryology* **Vol 1, Book 2** 193-205. Editor: Osborn, J.W.

Jones, S.J. and Boyde, A. 1974. Coronal cementogenesis in the horse. *Archives of Oral Biology* **19** 605-614.

Kaey, J.A. and Peek, J.M. 1980. Relationships between fires and winter habitat of deer in Idaho. *Journal of Wildlife Management* **44(2)** 372-380.

Kay, M. 1989. Prospects for archaeological seasonality estimates based on modern odocoileus virginianus cementum. Paper presented at the 54th annual meeting, Society for American Archaeology, Atlanta. April 5-9

Kay, M. 1974. Dental annuli age determination on White-tailed deer from archaeological sites. *Plains Anthropologist* **19(65)** 224-7.

Kay, R.F. and Cant, J.G.H. 1988. Age assessment using cementum annulus counts and tooth wear in a free-ranging population of maccaca mulatta. *American Journal of Primatology* **15** 1-15.

Kay, R.F., Rasmussen, D.T. and Beard, K.C. 1984. Cementum annulus counts provide a means for age determination in macca mulatta. *Folia Primatologica* **42** 85-95.

Kay, R.N.B. and Ryder, M.L. 1978. Coat growth in Red deer *(Cervus elephus)* exposed to a day-length cycle of six months duration. *Journal of Zoology Proceedings London* **185** 505.

Keiss, R.E. 1969. Comparison of eruption-wear patterns and cementum annuli as age criteria in elk. *Journal of Wildlife Management* **33** 175-80.

Kelly, R.L. 1983. Hunter-gatherer mobility strategies. *Journal of Anthropological Research* **39** 277-306.

Kerwin, M.L. and Mitchell, G.J. 1971. The validity of the wear-age technique for Alberta proghorns. *Journal of Wildlife Management* **35(4)** 743-747.

Kierdorf, U. and Becher, J. 1997. Mineralization and wear of mandibular first molars in Red deer *(Cervus elaphus)* of known age. *Journal of Zoology London* **241** 135-143.

Kierdorf, H. 1995. Determination of the season of death by cementum analysis on Reindeer teeth from Maszycka

Cave. *Maszyka Cave a Magdalenian site in Southern Poland.*

Klein, R.G. and Cruz-Urbibe, K. 1984. *The analysis of faunal remains from archaeological sites*. Chicago University Press

Klein, R.G., Wolf, C., Leslie, G. and Allwarden, K. 1981. The use of dental crown heights for constructing age profiles of Red deer and similar species in archaeological samples. *Journal of Archaeological Science* **8** 1-31.

Klein, R.G. and Cruz-Uribe, K. 1983. The computation of ungulate age (mortality) profiles from dental crown heights. *Palaeobiology* **9** 70-8.

Kleinenberg, S.E. and Klevezal, G.A. 1966. Age determination in mammals by the structure of tooth cement. *Zool.Zh* **45** 717-724.

Klevezal, G.A. 1980. Layers in the hard tissues of mammals as a record of growth rhythms of individuals. Growth of odontocetes and sirenians:problems in age determination *Proceedings of the Interernational.Conference on Determining Age of Odontocete Ceteans..La Jolla,California Sept 5-19* 1978 89-94. Cambridge International Whaling Commission

Klevezal, G.A. 1970. Retrospective evaluation of individual features of the growth of mammals by the layered structure of teeth and bone. *Ontogenez* **4** 362-372.

Klevezal, G.A. and Kleinenberg, S.E. 1967. *Age Determination of mammals from annual layers in teeth and bones*. Acadamy of Science USSR.Trans 1969 Dept.Interior & National Science Foundation, US Dept Commerce.

Klevezal, G.A., Sukhouskaya, L.I. and Kiseleva E.G. 1991. On sensitivity of dentine and cementum as recording structures using the example of deciduous and permanent teeth in bison. *Zool.Zh* **70:2** 119-126.

Klevezal, G.A.and Pucek, Z. 1987. Growth layers in tooth cement and dentine of European bison and its hybrids with domestic cattle. *Acta Theriologica* **32:9** 115-128.

Klevesal, G.A. 1996. *Recording structures of mammals. Determination of age and reconstruction of life history.* A.A. Balkema/Rotterdam/Brookfield.

Koch, P.L. and Fisher, D.C. 1989. Oxygen isotope variation in the tusks of extinct proboscidians:a measure of season of death and seasonality. *Geology* **17** 515-519.

Koike, H. 1979. Seasonal dating and the valve-pairing technique in shell-midden analysis. *Journal of Archaeological Science.* **6** 63-74.

Koike, H. and Ohtaishi, N. 1985. Prehistoric hunting pressure estimated by the age composition of excavated Sika deer *(Cervus nippon).* Using the annual layer of tooth cement. *Journal of Archaeological Science* **12** 443-456.

Koike, H. and Ohtaishi, N. 1985. Estimation of prehistoric hunting routes based on the age composition of Sika deer *(Cervus nippon). Journal of Archaeological Science* **14** 443-456.

Kolb, H. 1978. The formation of lines in the cementum of premolar teeth in foxes. *Journal of Zoology Society Zoology Proceedings London* **185** 259-263.

Korschgen, L.J., Porath, W.R. andTorgerson O. 1980. Spring and summer foods of deer in the Missouri. *Journal of Wildlife Management* **44(1)** 89-97.

Kozlowski, S.K. and Sachse-Kozlowska, E. 1993. Maszyka Cave a Magdalenian Site in Southern Poland.

Kubota, K., Matsumoto, K., Nagasaki, F. and Tsuboi, M. 1963. An age determination of the highly aged Fur seal by means of photography of the maxillary canine. *Bulletin of the Tokyo Medical and Dental University.* **10(1)** 61-73

Kvam, T. 1984. Age determination in European lynx *(Lynx L lynx)* by incremental lines in tooth cementum. *Acta Zool Fenn* **171** 73-75.

Landon, D.B. 1993. Testing a seasonal slaughter model for colonial New England using tooth cementum incremental analysis. *Journal of Archaeological Science* **20** 439-455.

Larson, J.S. and Taber, R.D. 1980. Criteria of sex and age. *Wildlife management technique manual* 143-202. The Wildlife Society

Laws, R.M. 1953. A new method of age determination in mammals with special reference to the Elephant seal *(Mirounga leonina). Scient.Rep.Falkld.Isl.Depend.Surv*. **2** 1-10.

Laws, R.M. 1952. A new method of age determination for mammals. *Nature.London* **169** 972-973.

Laws, R.M. 1960. Laminated structure of bones from some marine mammals. *Nature* **187** 338-339.

Leader-Williams, N. 1979. Age determination of Reindeer introduced into South Georgia. *Journal of Zoology London* **188** 501-15.

Legge, A.J. and Rowley-Conway, P.A. 1991. "Art made strong with bones": A review of some approaches to Osteoarchaeology. *International Journal of Osteoarchaeology* **1** 3-15.

Legge, A.J. and Rowley-Conway, P.A. 1988. *Star Carr revisited.* Birkbeck College

Levitan, B. 1982. Errors in recording tooth wear in ovicaprid mandibles at different speeds. Ageing and sexing animal bones from archaeological sites *BAR* **109** 223-250.

Lieberman, D.E. 1994. The biological basis for seasonal increments in dental cementum and their application to archaeological research. *Journal of Archaeological Science* **21** 525-539.

Lieberman, D.E. 1993. Life history variables preserved in dental cementum microstructure. *Science* **261** 1162-4.

Lieberman, D.E., Deacon, T.W. and Meadow R.H. 1990. Computer image enhancement and analysis of cementum increments as applied to teeth of *gazella gazella. Journal of Archaeological Science* **17** 519-533.

Lieberman, D.E. and Meadow, R.H. 1992. The biology of cementum increments with an archaeological application. *Mammal Review* **22:2** 57-77.

Lincoln, J.A. 1992. Biology of antlers. *Journal of Zoology London* **226** 517-528.

Linhart, S.B. and Knowlton, F.F. 1967. Determining age of coyotes by tooth cementum layers. *Journal of Wildlife Management* **31(2)** 362-5.

Lockard, G.R. 1972. Further studies of dental annuli for ageing White-tailed deer. *Journal of Wildlife Management* **36** 46-55.

Low, W.A. and Cowan, I.M. 1963. Age determination of deer by annular structure of dental cementum. *Journal of Wildlife Management* **27** 466-71.

Lowe, V.P.W. 1969. Population dynamics of the Red deer *(Cervus elaphus)* on Rhum. *Journal of Animal Ecology* **38** 425-457.

Lowe, V.P.W. 1967. Teeth as indicactors of age with special reference to Red deer *(Cervus elaphus)* of known age from Rhum. *Journal of Zoology London* **152** 137-53.

Lowenstam, H.A. and Weiner, S. 1989. *On Biomineralisation.* Oxford University Press.

Ludwig, T.G., Cuttress T.W. and Healy, W.B. 1966. Wear of sheep's teeth III. Seasonal variation in wear and ingested soil. *New Zealand Journal of Agricultural Research* **9** 157-64.

Madsen, R.M. 1967. Age determination of wildlife - a bibliography. Bibl #2. US Dept of the interior, dept lib, Washington

Magnaghi, N., Mendolia, C., Ferrante, V., Canali, V. and Carenzi, C. 1992. Behaviour of Red deer in a restricted area. *Journal of the British Deer Society* **8,8** 508-.

Mahoney, R. 1973. *Laboratory techniques in zoology.* **2nd edition** Butterworth,London.

Maltby, J.M. 1982. The variability of faunal samples and their effects on ageing data. *Ageing and sexing animal bones from archaeological sites BAR* **109** 81-90.

Mansfield, A.W. and Fisher, H.D. 1960. Age determination in the Harbour seal *(Phocavitulina L.).* Nature **186** 92-93.

Manson, R.A., Stone, W.B. and Parks, E. 1973. Ageing Red foxes *(Vulpes vulpes)* by counting the annular cementum rings of their teeth. *N.Y.Fish Game J.* **20** 54-61.

Marks, S.A. and Erickson, A.W. 1966. Age determination in the Black bear. *Journal of Wildlife Management* **30(2)** 389-.

Martin, H. 1994. *Nouveaux mileux, nouveaux chasseurs: une approche des comportements au post-glaciaire a` travers l'e'tude des saisons de capture du gibier*

Matson, G.M. 1989. Age Determination by tooth cementum analysis. Age data analysis. *Histology and Reproduction Studies.* **Progress report No 11** 1-8.

Matson, G.M. 1981. *Workbook for cementum analysis.* 1-30. Matson's Milltown, Montana

Matson, G.M. 1987. Matson's tooth cementum age analysis. . *Histology and Reproductive Studies.* **Progress Report No. 9** 1-7.

Matson, G.M. 1988. Tooth cementum age analysis. Data management and analysis. *Histology and Reproductive Studies.* **Progress Report No 10** 1-7.

Mayhew, D.F. 1978. Age structure of a sample of subfossil beavers *(Castor fiber L). Development, function and evolution of teeth* 495-505. Academic Press

Mays, S., Concepion de la Rue. and Molleson T. 1995. Molar crown height as a measure of evaluating existing dental wear scales for estimating age of death in human skeletal remains. *Journal of Archaeological Science* **22** 659-670.

McAlister, B., Miki, Y. and Norayanan, A.S. 1990. Isolation of a fibroblast attachment protein from cementum. *Journal of Periodontal Research* **25** 99-105.

McCance, R.A., Brown, W.A.B. and Ford, E.H.R. 1961. Severe undernutrition in growing and adult animals. *British Journal of Nutrition* **15** 213- 224.

McCullough, D.R. 1996. Failure of the tooth cementum ageing technique with reduced population density of deer. *Wildlife Society Bulletin 1996* **24(4)** 722-724.

McCutchen, H. 1969. Age determination of proghorns by the incisor cementum. *Journal of Wildlife Management* **33** 172-175.

McEwan, E.N. 1963. Seasonal annuli in the cementum of the teeth of Barren Ground caribou. *Canadian Journal of Zoology* **41** 111-113.

McLaren, I.A. 1958. The biology of the Ringed seal *(Phoca hispida Schreber)* in the Eastern Canadian Arctic. *Fisheries Research Board of Canada, Bulletin.* **118** Ottawa

McNally, L. 1975. *The year of the Red deer.* London.J.M.Dent & Sons

Mcneil, R.L. and Somerman, M.J. 1993. Molecular factors regulating development and regeneration of cementum. *Journal of Periodontal Research* **28:6.2** 550-559.

Meadow, R.H., Toplyn, M.R. and Gordon, B.C. 1989. An approach to the study of incremental structures. Paper presented at the 54th Annual meeting, Society for American archaeology, Atlant

Mellars, P.A. 1976. Fire, ecology, animal populations and man; a study of some ecological relationships in Prehistory. *Proceedings of the Prehistoric Society* **42** 15-45.

Miles, A.E.W. 1978. Teeth as an indicator of age in man. *Development, function and evolution of teeth* 455-464. Academic Press

Miller, F.L. 1974. Age determination of Caribou by annulations in dental cementum. *Journal of Wildlife Management* **38:1** 47-53.

Miller, F. 1974. Biology of the Kaminuriak population of Barren Ground Caribou Ottowa. part II. Dentition as an indicator of age and sex: composition and socialisation of the population. *Canadian Wildlife Service Reports* **31** 3-87.

Miller, F.L. 1972. Eruption and attrition of mandibular teeth in Barren-Ground Caribou. *Journal of Wildlife Management* **36:2** 602-612.

Mitchell, B. 1967. Growth layers in dental cement for determining the age of Red deer *(Cervus elephus L.). Journal of Animal Ecology* **36** 279-93.

Mitchell, B. 1963. Determination of age in Scottish Red deer from growth layers in dental cement. *Nature, London* **198** 350-351.

Mitchell, B. Determining the age of Red deer from growth layers in the dental cement. *Journal of the British Deer Society* 28-29.

Mitchell, B. Notes on two old Red deer. *Journal of the British Deer Society* 568-570.

Mitchell, B and Youngson, RW. *Teeth and age in Scottish Red deer a practical guide to age assessment.* The Red Deer Commission.

Molleson, T.I. and Cohen, P. 1990. The progression of dental attrition stages used for age assessment. *Journal of Archaeological Science* **17** 363-371.

Monks, G. 1981. Seasonality studies. *Advances in Archaeological Method and Theory* **4** 177-240. Academic Press, New York

Monks, G. and Johnston, R. 1993. Estimating season of death from growth increment data: a critical review. *Archaeozoologia* **5:2** 17-40.

Moore, N.P., Kelly, P.F., Hayden, T.J. and Cahill, P.F. 1995. An assessment of five methods of age determination in an enclosed population of Fallow deer *(Dama dama). Biology and Environment: Proceedings of the Royal Irish Academy* **95B** 1 27-34.

Morris, P. 1978. The use of teeth for estimating the age of wild animals. *Development, function and evolution of teeth* 483-94. Academic Press, New York

Morris, P.A. 1972. A review of mammalian age determination methods. *Mammal Review* **2:3** 69-104.

Morris, P.A. 1970. A method for determining absolute age in the hedgehog. *Journal of Zoology London* **161(2)** 277-281.

Mundy, K.R.D. and Fuller, W.A. 1964. Age determination in the Grizzly bear. *Journal of Wildlife Management* **28** 863-866.

Munson, P.J. 1984. Teeth of juvenile woodchuck as seasonal indicators on archaeological sites. *Journal of Archaeological Science* **11** 395-403.

Myric, A.C. 1980. Examination of layered tissue of Odontocetes for age determination using polarized lightmicroscopy. *Age determination of Toothed Whales and Sirenians* 105-112. Cambridge.

Nalbabion, J. and Frank, R.M. 1980. Electron microscopic study of the regeneration of cementum and periodontal connective tissue in the cat. *Journal of Periodontal Research* **15** 71-89.

Narayanan, S.A. and Yonemura, K. 1993. Purification and characterisation of a novel growth factor from cementum. *Journal of Periodontal Research* **28:6.2** 563-565.

Naylor, J.W., Stokes G.N. and Miller, W.G. 1985. Cementum annulation enhancement: a technique for age determination in man. *American Journal of Physical Anthropology* **68** 197-200.

Noe-Nygaard, N. 1983. A new find of Brown bear *(Ursus arctos)* from Star Carr and other finds in the late glacial and post glacial of Britain and Denmark. *Journal of Archaeological Science* **10** 317-325.

Noe-Nygaard, N. 1975. Two shoulder blades with healed lesions from Star Carr. *Proceedings of the Prehistoric Society* **41** 10-16.

Noe-Nygaard, N. 1974. Mesolithic hunting in Denmark illustrated by bone injuries caused by human weapons. *Journal of Archaeological Science* **1** 217-248.

Noe-Nyggard, N. 1977. Butchering and marrow fracturing as a taphonomic factor in archaeological deposits. *Paleobiology* **3** 218-237.

Noodle, B. 1982. The size of Red deer in Britain - past and present, with some reference to Fallow deer. **146** *Archaeological aspects of woodland ecology* 315-328.

Novakowski, N.S. 1965. Cementum deposition as an age criterion in Bison and the relation of incisor wear, eye-lens weight and dressed carcass weight to age. *Canadian Journal of Zoology* **43:1** 173-178.

Nudds, T.D. 1980. Forage preference: Theoretical considerations of diet selection by deer. *Journal of Wildlife Management* **44(3)** 735-739.

O'Brien, C. 1994. Determining seasonality and age in East African archaeological faunas:an ethnoarchaeological application of cementum increment analysis. *PhD thesis*, University of Wisconsin, Madison. University Microfilms, Ann Arbor, Michigan.

Ohtaishi, N., Miura, S., Wu, J. and Kaji, K. 1990. Age determination of the White lipped deer *(Cervus albirostris)* by dental cementum and molar wear. *Journal-Mammal-Soc-JPN* **15:1** 25-24.

Ohtaishi, N. 1980. Determination of sex, age and death season of recovered remains of Sika deer *(Cervus Nippon)* by jaw and tooth cement. *Kokogaku to Shizenkagaku* **13** 51-73.

Olsen. S.L. 1988. Applications of scanning electron microscopy to archaeology *BAR. International Series* **452**

Omar, S. 1992. Ageing deer from cementum bands. *Journal of the British Deer Society* **8:9** 569-572.

Osborn, J.W. 1981. *Dental anatomy and embryology.* Oxford. Blackwell Scientific

Pantin, C.F.A. 1959. *Notes on microscopical technique for zoologists.* Cambridge University Press

Parkin, R.A., Serjeantson, D. and Rowley-Conway, P. 1986. Late Paleolithic exploitation of horse and Red deer at Gough's Cave Cheddar, Somerset. *Proceedings of the University of Bristol Speleological Society* **17** 311-330.

Pawley, J.B. 1995. *Handbook of Biological Confocal Microscopy.* Plenum Press, New York

Payne, S. 1987. Reference codes for wear states in the mandibular cheek teeth of sheep and goats. *Journal of Archaeological Science* **14** 14.

Payne, S. 1973. Kill off patterns in sheep and goats: The mandibles from Asvan Kale. *Anatolian Studies* **23** 281-303.

P'erez-Barberia, F.J. 1994. Determination of age in Cantabrian Chamois *(Rupicapa pyrenaica parua)* from jaw tooth row eruption and wear. *Journal of Zoology London* **233** 649-656.

Pike-Tay, A. 1991. L'Analyse du cement dentire chez les cerfs: L'application en prehistoire. *Paleo* **3** 149-166.

Pike-Tay, A. and Bricker, H.M. 1993. Hunting in the Gravettian: an examination of evidence from South Western France. *Arch.papers of the American Anthropological Association* **4** 127-143.

Pike-Tay, A. 1991. Red deer hunting in the Upper Paleolithic of South West France: a study in seasonality. *B.A.R.(International series)* **569**

Pike-Tay, A. 1995. Variability and synchrony of seasonal indicators in dental cementum microstructure of the Kaminuriak Caribou population. *Archaeofauna.* **4**

Pike-Tay, A. 1993. Hunting in the Upper Perigordian: a matter of strategy or expedience? *Before Lascaux: The complex record of the Early Upper Paleolithic.* CRC Press,Boca Raton.

Pitts, M. 1979. Hides and antlers: a new look at the gatherer-hunter site at Star Carr, North Yorkshire, England. *World Archaeology* **11/1** 32-42.

Pogge, F.L. 1967. Elm as deer browse. *Journal of Wildlife Management* **31(2)** 354-356.

Pollitt, E.A. 1993. Age related incremental growth patterns in cementum. *Unpublished dissertation University of Wales.*

Pollock, A.M. 1975. Seasonal changes in appetite and sexual condition in Red deer stags maintained on a six-month photoperiod. *Journal .Physiol.Lond* **244** 95-96.

Presley, S. 1987. Determination of site seasonality using tooth annulus technique. Archaeology Survey of Canada Archives. Ottawa Hull.

Price, T.D. 1982. Willow tales and dog smoke. *Quarterly Review of Archaeology*. 3pp, not numbered.

Prior, R. 1968. *The Roe deer of Cranbourne Chase.* Oxford: University Press.

Putman, R.J. and Hunt, E.J. 1993. Hybridisation between Red and Sika deer in Britain. *Journal of the British Deer Society* **9:2**

Quere, J.P. and Pascal, M. 1983. Comparaison de plusieurs methodes de la determination d'age individuel chez le cerf elaphe *(Cervus elephus L)*. Annables des Sciences Naturelles Zoologie **13(5)** 235-252.

Quimby, D.C. and Gaab, J.E. 1957. Mandibular dentition as an age indicator in Rocky Mountain Elk. *Journal of Wildlife Management* **21:4** 435-451.

Raesfeld von, F. 1971. *Das Rotwild.* Hamburg & Berlin

Raesfeld von, F. and Vorreyer, F. 1978. *Das Rotwild.* Hamburg & Berlin

Ransome, A.B. 1966. Determining age of the White-tailed deer from layers in cementum of molars. *Journal of Wildlife Management* **30(1)** 197-9.

Ratcliffe, P.R. and Mayle, B.A. 1992. Roe deer biology and management. *Bulletin **105*** Forestry Commission

Ratcliffe, P.R. 1987. The management of Red deer in upland forests. *Bulletin **71*** Forestry Commission

Reimers, E. and Norby, O. 1968. Relationship between age and tooth cementum layers in Norwegian Reindeer. *Journal of Wildlife Management* **32(4)** 957-961.

Rice, L.A. 1980. Influences of irregular dental cementum layers on ageing deer incisors. *Journal of Wildlife Management* **44(1)** 266-268.

Riney, T. 1951. Standard terminology for deer teeth. *Journal of Wildlife Management* **15(1)** 99-101.

Roberts, J.D. 1978. Variation in coyote age determination from annuli in different teeth. *Journal of Wildlife Management* **42** 454-456.

Robinette, W.L., Rogers, G., Gashwiler, J.S. and Jones, D.A. 1957. Notes on tooth development and wear for Rocky Mountain Mule deer. *Journal of Wildlife Management* **21(2)** 134-153.

Robinette, W.L. and Archer, A.L. 1971. Notes on ageing criteria and reproduction of Thomson's gazelle. *East African Wildlife Journal* **9** 83-99.

Rogers, L.L., Dawson, D.K. and Mech, L.D. 1980. Deer distribution in relation to wolf pack territory edges. *Journal of Wildlife Management* **44(1)** 253-257.

Rose, H. 1994. Scottish deer distribution survey. *Journal of the British Deer Society* **9,3** 153-156.

Rose, H. 1989. Winter mortality in Scotland. *Journal of the British Deer Society* **7:9**

Rowley-Conwy, P. 1995. Mesolithic settlement patterns: new zooarchaeological evidence from the Vale of Pickering, Yorkshire. *University of Durham & University of Newcastle upon Tyne Archaeological Reports* 19941 - 7.

Rudge, M.R. 1976. Ageing domestic sheep *(Ovis aries L)* from growth lines in the cementum of the first incisor. *New Zealand Journal of Zoology* **3** 421-424.

Sauer, P. 1973. Seasonal variation in physiology of White-tailed deer in relation to cementum annulus formation. *PhD dissertation*, State University of New York at Albany.

Sauer, P.F. 1971. Tooth sectioning versus tooth wear for assigning age to White-tailed deer. *Trans.Northeast Fish and Wildlife Conference*. **28** 9-20.

Savelle, J.M. and Albright, D. 1989. Comparison of preparation and examination techniques in dental annuli analysis. Paper presented at the 54th Annual meeting, Society for American Archaeology.Atlanta April 5-9

Savelle, J. and Beattie, O. 1983. Analysis of dental annuli in Muskoxen *(Ovibos moshalus)* as an aid in the determination of archaeological site seasonality. *Canadian Journal of Anthropology* **3:1** 123-129.

Saville, J. and Will, R. 1982. Dental annuli analysis as an aid in the determination of copper inuit subsistence strategies. Paper presented at the 15th Annual meeting of the Canadian Archaeological Association, Hamilton.

Saxon, A. and Higham, C.F.W. 1968. Identification and interpretation of growth rings in the secondary cementum of Ovis aries L. *Nature,London* **219** 634-5.

Saxon, A. and Higman, C. 1968. A new research method for economic prehistorians. *American Antiquity* **34(3)** 303-311.

Schadla-Hall, R.T. 1988. The early post glacial in eastern Yorkshire. *Archaeology in Eastern Yorkshire; Essays in honour of TCM Brewster* 25-34.

Scheffer, V.B. 1950. Growth layers on the teeth of Pinnipedia as an indication of age. *Science* **112** 309-311.

Schmidt, W.J. and Keil, A. 1972. *Polaizing microscopy of dental tissues.* Oxford:Pergaman Press

Schmidt, W.J. and Keil, A. 1971. *Polarizing microscopy.* Oxford:Pergaman Press

Schultz, V. 1967. Calcium content of White-tailed deer mandibles. *Journal of Wildlife Management* **31(3)** 591-593.

Scott, J.H. and Symons, N.B.B. 1974. *Introduction to dental anatomy.* 7th **edition** Churchill Livingstone, Edinburgh.

Sergeant, D.E. 1967. Age determination of land mammals from annuli. *Z.Seitschift fin Sauge trer Kunde. Dtsch* **32:5** 297-300.

Sergeant, D.E. and Pimlott, D.H. 1959. Age determination in Moose from sectioned incisor teeth. *Journal of Wildlife Management* **23:3** 315-321.

Sergeant, D.E. 1967. Age determination of land mammals from annuli. *Z-Seitschift fin Sauge her?? Kunde dtsh* **35(5)** 297-300.

Severinghaus, C.W. 1949. Tooth Development and wear as criteria of age in White-tailed deer. *Journal of Wildlife Management* **13** 195-216.

Shackleton, N.J. 1973. Oxygen isotope analysis as a means of determining season of occupation of prehistoric midden sites. *Archaeometry* **15 (1)** 133-141.

Shapiro, A.H. 1995. A study of cement layering in cattle teeth with a review of methods of age and season of death determination used in Zooarchaeology. *Unpublished MSc dissertation UCL*

Sherlock, M.G. and Fairly, J.S. 1993. Seasonal changes in the diet of Red deer *(Cervus elaphus)* in the Connemara National Park. *Biology and Environment* **9313(2)** 85-90.

Shiffer, M.B. 1976. *Behavioural archaeology.* Academic Press New York.

Sibbald, A.M., Kerr, W.G., Loudon, A.S.I. and Fenn, P.D. 1993. The influence of birth date on the development of seasonal cycles in Red deer hinds *(Cervus elaphus). Journal of Zoology (London)* **230(4)** 593-607.

Simkiss, K. 1975. *Bone and biomineralisation.* Camelot Press London

Simmons, I.G. 1979. Late mesolithic societies and the environment of the uplands of England and Wales. *Bulletin of the Institute of Arch* **16** 111-129.

Simmons, I.G. 1975. Towards an ecology of Mesolithic man in the uplands of Great Britain. *Journal of Archaeological Science* **4** 1-15.

Simmons, I.G. and Innes, J.B. 1987. Mid-holocene adaptations and later Mesolithic forest disturbance in Northern England. *Journal of Archaeological Science* **14** 385-403.

Simmons, I.G. 1996. *The environmental impact of later Mesolithic cultures.* Edinburgh University Press

Smith, R. 1970. An accurate ageing method for Elk. *Wildlife Digest, Arizona* **Abstract 5**

Smith, K.G. and Strother, J.C. 1994. Chemical ultrastructure of cementum growth layers of teeth of Black bears. *Journal of Mammal* **75(2)** 406-409.

Smuts, G.L., Austin, J.C. and Anderson, J.L. 1978. Age determination of the African lion (Panthera leo). *Journal of Zoology London* **185** 115-146.

Sohn, A.J. 1968. An evaluation of the demtal annuli technique for determining age of White-tailed deer in Iowa. *Iowa Academy of Science.* **74** 72-77.

Solhiem, T. 1990. Dental cementum apposition as an indicator of age. *Scan.J.Dent Res* **98:6** 510-519.

Solounias, N. and Hayek, L.A.C. 1993. New methods of tooth microwear analysis and application to dietry determination of two extinct antelopes. *Journal of Zoology London* **229** 421-45.

Sorensen, K.A. 1983. An example of taphonomic loss in a Mesolithic faunal assemblage. *BAR International* **163** 243-247

Speth, J.D. and Spielmann, K. 1983. Energy source, protein metabolism and hunter/gatherer subsistence strategies. *Journal of Anthropological Archaeology* **2** 1-3.

Spiess, A. 1989. Deer tooth sectioning, eruption, and seasonality of deer hunting in prehistoric Maine. Paper given at the 54th annual meeting of the Society for American Archaeology Atlanta.

Spiess, A. 1985. Deer tooth sectioning and seasonality of deer hunting at the Turner farm: 4500-1000 BP. Paper given at the 84th annual meeting of the American Anthropological Association, Washington

Spiess, A. 1979. *Reindeer and Caribou hunters: An archaeological study.* Academic Press, New York

Spiess, A. 1976. Determining season of death of archaeological fauna by analysis of teeth. *Artic* **29(1)** 23-55.

Spinage, C.A. 1976. Incremental cementum lines in the teeth of tropical African mammals. *Journal of Zoology London* **178** 117-131.

Spinage, C.A. 1973. A review of the age determination of mammals by means of teeth, with special reference to Africa. *East Africa Wildlife Journal* **11** 165-187.

Spinage, C.A. 1976. Age determination of the female Grant's gazelle. *East African Wildlife Journal* **14** 121-134.

Spinage, C.A. and Brown, W.A.B. 1988. Age determination of the West African Buffalo *(Syncerus caffer brachyceros)* and the constancy of tooth wear. *African Journal of Ecology* **26** 221-227.

Spinage, C.A. 1967. Ageing the Uganda Defassa Waterbuck *(Kobus defassa ugandae Neumann). East African Wildlife Journal* **5** 1-17.

Spurr, A.R. 1969. A low-viscosity epoxy resin embedding medium for electron microscopy. *Journal of Ultrastructure Research* **26** 31-43.

Staines, B.W. 1976. The use of natural shelter by Red deer in relation to weather in North East Scotland. *Journal of Zoology London* **180** 1-8.

Staines, B.W. and Crisp, J.M. 1978. Observations on food quality in Scottish Red deer *(Cervus elephus)* as determined by chemical analysis of the rumen contents. *Journal of Zoological Society. Zoology Proceedings London* **185** 253.

Stallibrass, S. 1982. The use of cementum layers for absolute ageing of mammalian teeth: a selective review of the literature, with suggestions for further studies and alternative applications. Ageing and sexing animal bones from archaeological sites *BAR International Series* **109** 109-126.

Steenkamp, J.D.G. 1975. Guidelines to the use of dental histology in wildlife research. *Journal of South African Wildlife Management Association* **5(2)** 89-94.

Stevens, M.L. 1983. A reliable celloidin technique for dental cementum analysis: a comment. *Journal of Wildlife Management* **47:4** 1243.

Stoddart, D. 1974. Age determination of Roe deer *(Capreolus capreolus)* from annular growth layers in dental cementum. *Journal of Zoology (London)* **174(4)** 511-537.

Stoneberg, R. and Jonkel, C. 1966. Age determination of Black bears by cementum layers. *Journal of Wildlife Management* **30:2** 411-4.

Stormer, F.A. and Bauer, W.A. 1980. Summer forage use by tame deer in Northern Michigan. *Journal of Wildlife Management* **44(1)** 98-106.

Stott, G.G., Levy, B.M., and Sis, R.F. 1982. Cementum annulation as an age criterion in forensic dentistry. *Journal of Dental Research* **61** 814-817.

Strandgaard, H. 1967. Reliability of the Petersen method tested on a Roe deer population. *Journal of Wildlife Management* **31(4)** 643-651.

Street, M. 1991. Bedburg-Konigshoven: a pre-boreal Mesolithic site in the Rhineland, Germany. The Late Glacial in north-west Europe:human adaptation and environmental change at the end of the Pleistocene. *CBA Research Report* **77** 256-270

Ten Cate, A.R. 1989. *Oral histology development, structure, and function.*The C.V.Mosby Co. Toronto

Thomas, D.C. 1977. Metachromatic staining of dental cementum for mammalian age determination. *Journal of Wildlife Management* **41** 207-11.

Thomas, D.C. and Bandy, P.J. 1973. Age determination of wild Black tailed deer from dental annulations. *Journal of Wildlife Management* **37** 232-235.

Thomas, D.C. and Bandy, P.J. 1975. Accuracy of dental-wear age estimates of Black tailed deer. *Journal of Wildlife Management* **39** 674-678.

Totdal, B. and Hals, E. 1985. Electron probe study of human and Red deer cementum and root dentine. *Scand.J.Dent.Res.* **93**:1 4-12.

Tumilson, R. and McDaniel, V.R. 1983. A reliable celloidin technique for dental cementum analysis. *Journal of Wildlife Management* **47:1** 274-278.

Tumlison, R. and McDaniel, V.R. 1983. A reliable celloidin technique for dental cementum analysis:a reply. *Journal of Wildlife Management* **47:4** 1244-1245.

Turner, J.C. 1977. Cemental annulations as an age criterion in North American sheep. *Journal of Wildlife Management* **41:2** 211-217.

van Nostrand, F.C. and Stephenson, A.B. 1964. Age determination for Beavers by tooth development. *Journal of Wildlife Management* **28** 430-4.

Wagenknecht, E. 1981. *Rotwild.* Neudamn

Walker, D. 1950. Second interim report on peat stratigraphy and pollen analysis in the Seamer area. *Proceedings of the Prehistoric Society* **16** 120-122.

Watson, A. and Staines, B.W. 1978. Differences in the quality of wintering areas used by male and female Red deer *(Cervus elaphus)* in Aberdeenshire Scotland UK. *Journal of Zoology London* **186:4** 544-550.

Welch, D., Catt, D.C., Scott, D. and Staines, B.W. 1990. Habitat usage by Red *(Cervus-elaphus)* and Roe *(Capreolus-capreolus)* deer in a Scottish spruce plantation. *Journal of Zoology London* **221:3** 453-476.

Wheeler, A. 1978. Why are there no fish remains at Star Carr? *Journal of Archaeological Science* **5** 85-90.

White, G. 1974. Age determination of Roe deer *(Capreolus-capreolus)* from annual growth layers in dental cementum. *Journal of Zoology London* **175:1** 15-28.

Willey, C.H. 1974. Ageing Black bears from first premolar tooth sections. *Journal of Wildlife Management* **38** 97-100.

Wilson, M. 1978. Cementum annuli in mammal teeth from archaeological sites. *Science* **202** 541-542.

Wolfe, M.L. 1969. Age determination in moose from cemental layers of molar teeth. *Journal of Wildlife Management* **33** 428-31.

Youngson, R. 1990. Red deer counts. *Journal of the British Deer Society* **8:1**

Youngson, R.W. 1970. Rearing Red deer calves in captivity. *Journal of Wildlife Management* **34:2** 466-70.

Zander, H.A. and Hürzeler, B. 1958. Continuous cementum apposition. *Journal of Dental Research* **37** 1035-44.